Aug

Dear Fortunée

It is with great pleasure that I share with you my personal true story.
I hope that you will enjoy.
With love
Nechama

The Will To Live

Nechama Surik

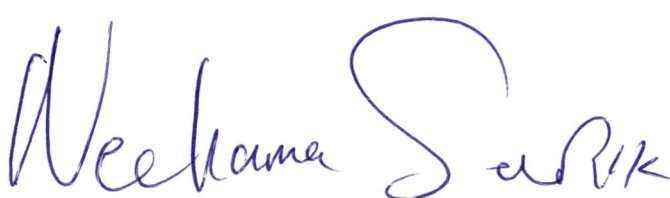

authorHOUSE

AuthorHouse™
1663 Liberty Drive, Suite 200
Bloomington, IN 47403
www.authorhouse.com
Phone: 1-800-839-8640

© *Nechama Surik. All Rights Reserved.*

No part of this book may be reproduced, stored in a retrieval system, or transmitted by any means without the written permission of the author.

First published by AuthorHouse 4/24/2009

ISBN: 978-1-4389-0946-2 (sc)
ISBN: 978-1-4389-0947-9 (hc)

Library of Congress Control Number: 2009901112

Printed in the United States of America
Bloomington, Indiana

This book is printed on acid-free paper.

nechama@nechamasurik.com

*This book is dedicated with love to the greatest heroes I have ever known:
My parents*

FRIDA and MEIR SURIK

Editor:
Edwin Orion Brownell

Translation from Hebrew:
Michal Rosenbaum
Shiri Rosenbaum

Cover page painting:
Antoinette Brownell

Cover page photography:
Yakov Cohen

Acknowledgements

This book began as a journal written for my father. When the words were first set to paper, publishing was not even a dream, let alone my original intention. However, after long consideration, I began to think of how my family's story and the heroism of my mom and dad could inspire others facing similar difficulties. As Canada faces its own health care crisis, I realized that both our positive and negative experiences with the Israeli system were worth recounting as well.

This book is the result and while its faults are my responsibility, its success is due to the help of my beloved family and my many dear friends.

To my two beloved and beautiful daughters, **Michal** and **Shiri**, I send my love and heartfelt thanks for your wonderful translation, your continuous love, and your steadfast support. You have matured into wonderful women and are my greatest source of pride and inspiration. **I love you.**

My deepest thanks go to the love of my life, **Edwin Orion Brownell**; without your support, help, and daily encouragement, this book could not have been published. Thank you for the most beautiful editing and for the many months of hard work you have put into this book. Above all, Edwin, I thank you for the joy, love, and new meaning you brought into my life. My heart and love are yours forever.

I am filled with happiness to have the beautiful artwork of **Mrs. Antoinette Brownell**, Edwin's mom (or, as we call her, MeeMee), appearing on the cover of my book. I feel very fortunate and proud to have your work adorning The Will To Live, and I send you my heartfelt thanks for this wonderful gift.

My love and gratitude to my three brothers and their wives: Yehuda and Aviva Surik, Raffi and Ayelet Surik, Yossi and Keren Surik. Your boundless dedication and care gave Mom and Dad the **will to live**; without you they would not have survived.

To Michal, Shiri, Yaniv, Sivan, Danielle, Gali, Yuval, and Kfir: you are the light, the joy, and the hope in Grandma and Grandpa's lives each and every day.

I send my heartfelt thanks to David Rosenbaum, for his assistance during the troubled times of my father's injury.

To my uncle and aunt, Israel and Chaviva Baron, to Shimon and Niuta Kutchinsky, to Rachel and Moshe Melnick, and to the entire extended family and friends – our deep gratitude for supporting my parents.

My special thanks and everlasting love to Orit and Eitan Ariel, my beloved friends. You are more than my friends - you are my family.

To Jacques Forest, thank you for being a wonderful friend and a daily source of comfort.

I give my thanks to my colleague Dr. Jack Gaiptman, who offered his help on several matters. Assistant Professor in the Department of Family Medicine of McGill University, Chief Attending Physician at Maimonides Geriatric Centre in Montreal, and family doctor at the Clinique Medicale Ville Emard, Dr. Gaiptman is an exceptional physician who is also known for his great sense of humor. I offer you my deep gratitude for all your assistance.

I would like to extend my thanks to Sharonne Cohen for all her professional help.

The management of Maimonides Geriatric Hospital has provided me with real and consistent support in personal matters as well as in regards to my professional development. I thank you all with my whole heart for the understanding and generosity you have always shown.

Last but not least, I send my gratitude to the staff of the Ichilov Medical Center in Tel Aviv and the Beith Rivka Rehabilitation Center in Petach Tikva. Because of your care, dedication, and devotion, our father is alive. I thank you on behalf of my entire family.

Preface

The Will to Live is a true, personal story. The names, dates, and details mentioned in the book are all factual.

In the year 2000, my father was injured in a near-fatal car accident. His life was altered forever in a fraction of a moment, as were the lives of his family members.

This book is about an honest, hard-working man's struggle to live. It also describes the many complex dilemmas and the moral and ethical questions our family was forced to deal with, none of which had clear-cut answers. As an RNA (Registered Nursing Assistant), I naturally confronted these issues from two perspectives: the professional and the personal. My work depends on the training and the experience I have gained over the years, and – as importantly – on my intuition, my values, and my conscience. I acquired my nursing license in Canada, never having practiced in Israel, so my father's injury was my introduction as a professional to the Israeli health system. This made me aware of the similarities and differences between the Israeli and Canadian models – particularly in terms of the medical professionals' attitudes and regarding technological aspects of treatment.

While I learned much about Israeli health care throughout the time of my father's recovery, I learned even more about our human reactions to crisis.

This is the story of my family, our friends, and the people we encountered at such a time. It is also the story of how the will to live can overcome any obstacle we face.

A Brief Introduction to the Family

My dear parents, Frida and Meir, were married on November 5, 1957, in Neve Monosson, a community in central Israel. Their wedding remains etched in the memory of the community's long-standing members, as my parents were the first to be married there, in the presence of its founder, Ephraim (Fred) Monosson.

Ephraim Monosson was a Jewish-American Zionist who saw the need to establish a community close to Ben Gurion airport in Tel Aviv. This would serve as a convenient and accessible place of residence for the airport's employees. Thanks to his vision, and an extremely generous monetary donation, the cornerstone of Neve Monosson was laid in December 1953, and its settlement began in 1955. The neighborhood was unique in that only private homes were built within its perimeters; permits were not granted to construct high-rises. Many of the workers employed at the airport began purchasing houses, and the village quickly grew, gaining the reputation of a prestigious, exclusive community.

* * *

My father, Meir Surik, was born in Poland in 1930. After experiencing many of the hardships that befell his fellow Eastern-Europeans in the 1930s and 40s, he came alone, without papers or identification, via a difficult, circuitous route, to British Mandate Palestine as part of the 1946 wave of illegal immigration. Upon arrival, he was given two Liras (currency, equivalent to a few cents) by the Jewish Immigration Agency, and that, with the clothes on his back and a determination to make a life for himself in his new homeland, was all he had.

While still in Europe, Dad joined the Haganah,[1] underwent training and served as a youth instructor and counselor. He planned to join the army once he got to Palestine, but being sixteen years old on his arrival, discovered that he could not enlist, as official recruitment only began at eighteen. My father took advantage of the fact that he had no identification papers and declared that he was of age (born January 1st, 1928) though he was actually born two years later. This falsehood has remained with him throughout his life, as it is the date registered on his ID card. So at

---

[1] The Haganah was the defense force of the Jewish community and the Zionist movement prior to the establishment of the state of Israel.

sixteen, Dad was drafted into the army, and given substantial responsibility, transformed from a child to a proud soldier overnight.

When my father departed for Palestine, he left behind his mother, his married sister, her husband, and her infant son. He had no idea what had become of them. Two weeks after his arrival, he met a soldier who had known his family in Europe, who told Dad he was convinced he had seen the entire family at an immigrant camp in Pardes Hanna, south of Haifa. Thrilled and excited to hear the news, my father immediately asked his commander to approve a leave of absence so he could find them. His commander refused, claiming that the following morning their unit was to set out for the Negev, the desert in the south of Palestine. Dad, a child-soldier, had no intention of postponing his unification with his loved ones for even one moment. He insisted on going, explaining to his commander that rather than having a defector on his hands, he'd be better off approving the leave and having him back at the base the following morning. Finally the commander gave in and reluctantly agreed. Several hours later my dad found his family, and after a short but emotional reunion, kept his promise to return to the base on time.

My grandmother, Zina Surik, was a strong woman who devoted her entire life to our family. My aunt, Rivka Melnik, Dad's sister, was also very special. Together with my father and Uncle Zeev, they started adjusting to Israel, and after my grandmother began working for El Al (the Israeli national airline), they were able to purchase a home in Neve Monosson. Aunt Rivka raised her family there, as did my parents.

Grandma, who was widowed at an early age while still in Europe, never remarried. She lived with us and lovingly devoted her life to her children, grandchildren, and great-grandchildren. While often criticized for her toughness and her need to dominate and control the family's dynamics, Grandma, or *Babbe*, as she was referred to by all her grandchildren, was a motherly, caring, protective, warm, and loving woman. Her dedication to the family was never questioned, and our love for her is eternal.

When I was eleven or twelve years old, I shared a very special time alone with my Babbe. Every week, Friday evening was "our time." On this night, Israeli TV played an Arabic movie. While these movies were for our Arab population and had no subtitles, they were still wildly popular throughout Israel. They were known for their cheesy love stories, their music, and their over-the-top drama, much as "Bollywood" Indian cinema is famous for today. We used to get ready half an hour before "show time," making tea and preparing the cake that went with it. Then, as we watched the film, I used to "translate" the story for Babbe. Of course I never spoke Arabic, but I made up my own story as the action unfolded on the screen. I would get into the characters and not only explain what they were saying but act out what I was seeing. She used to adore this and said that my interpretation was probably better than the original. It was a very high-pressure situation, but I loved my role! My grandmother enjoyed these evenings so much that she once wrote a letter to the TV station, requesting the Arabic movies more often..

My aunt Rivka was a beloved and strong figure in our family. She died of cancer at a relatively young age, only a few years after the passing of her husband, Zeev. Her death was a severe blow, as she was the link connecting all of us. Her home was always welcoming, her door was always open, and I miss her tremendously. While her children, my cousins, live in Neve Monosson to this day, I am sad to say that since Aunt Rivka's passing we see each other only at funerals and other significant family events.

* * *

My mother, Frida, who was also born in Poland, grew up in Russia and came to Israel much later than my father. My maternal grandfather had died when Mom was very young, but the rest of the family stuck together on the long journey to Israel. Frida arrived on April 16, 1957, together with her mother, Luba Vinrich (*Babba Luba*), her brother Israel, and his father, my mom's beloved stepfather, Moishe. This was a historic date for my mother and our entire family, and not just because it was her eighteenth birthday, the eve of Passover, and their first time setting foot in the land of Israel. On the very same evening, this beautiful, excited, and exhausted young woman met the man with whom she'd spend the rest of her life: my father.

Dad was sent to welcome her at the seaport as a friend of a relative. By a happy twist of fate, as she was walking down the gangplank exiting the ship, my father was the first person she would meet in her new homeland.

I had not given this encounter much consideration until I began writing this memoir, and only now do I realize how exceptional and romantic it was.

My father, the young suitor, immediately took upon himself the responsibility of looking after my mother's acclimation, as he was already an "old timer" by then. He registered Mom at an Ulpan[2] in Kibbutz[3] Sdot Yam, and took care of all the necessary arrangements. He also found a practical way to win the heart of the most beautiful woman he had ever met. Many of you are

---

[2] An Ulpan is a Hebrew language class.

[3] The Kibbutzim are the communities originally settled by Eastern European immigrants to Israel that are primarily agricultural in nature and based on a system of collective ownership. Many still exist today, although they operate from more capitalistic foundations.

no doubt familiar with suitors calling on young ladies with a beautiful bouquet of flowers, a delicious bottle of champagne, some fragrant perfume, or a piece of jewelry. Well, *my* father decided to be original; once he discovered that my mother was crazy about cold cuts, he used to pick out fine meats at the delicatessen and rush over to visit his beloved. The tactic paid off; my parents wed, and they are still happily married. On November 5, 2007, they commemorated their fiftieth wedding anniversary with a big, emotional party. Relatives from across Israel and North America attended this celebration of their love.

The first five years of my parents' marriage were years of painful adaptation, particularly due to the serious illnesses that struck both of them. Dad contracted an extremely aggressive Meningitis infection, and the doctors gave him little chance of surviving. Mom was already carrying their first child, and the family spent a long period of time in fear for his life. However, the infection was eventually beaten, the will to live triumphed, and Dad recovered completely.

Several months after the birth of my older brother Yehuda in 1958, the family was staggered by yet another blow: Mom had contracted tuberculosis. In the 1950s, it was one of those "shameful" illnesses that no one talked about, being highly contagious and life-threatening, and to this day she has never liked discussing it. My mother's hospitalization was another time of crisis, in part from natural fears for her health but also from complex family dynamics. While she became very ill, our extended family rallied around, and with their financial and emotional support the healing process began, and my mother pulled through.

Dad began working in the field of building insulation. He worked untiringly and quickly advanced to the position of production manager, eventually becoming a key figure in every company he worked for. His job required lots of traveling to distant locations, and this only allowed him home for weekends. We, the children, never complained; accustomed to his schedule, we knew no other. Every Friday, as everyone was busy preparing for Dad's homecoming, we'd feel a sense of anticipation for his arrival. You could smell it in the air, as the scents of cooking and baking filled the house with delicious aromas. Just before Dad would come, we'd wait on the balcony for the sight of his car, and as it appeared, we would all run downstairs to jump on him shouting: "Abbalee Abbalee (Daddy, Daddy)!" Every weekend was so special for us, and we usually spent the time celebrating with family and close friends. Whether home or out visiting, I especially enjoyed the company of the Feldstein and Bazostek families.

Chaim Feldstein was a friend of Dad's back in Europe. When he moved to Israel he built a home in a town northeast of Haifa with his wife Bruria and their three children.

Chaim's son Yossi, a paratrooper, was killed in a tragic helicopter accident during training. Our families were so close that when my youngest brother was born a few months later, he was named after him. The friendship between Chaim and Dad was indeed as thick as blood, and although he recently passed away following a long illness, he leaves behind many wonderful memories forever treasured in our hearts.

Shoshana Bzostek, my father's cousin, and her husband, Moishe, lived near Tel Aviv for many years, then moved across the ocean to New York. During their time in Israel, the ties between our two families were tight. We spent a great deal of time enjoying nature with them – having picnics in the forests of Ben Shemen and picking mushrooms there in the early morning following the Yoree, the first rain of the Israeli winter. At six in the morning we'd put on high rubber boots, take plastic baskets to hold our fresh mushrooms, and head out for adventure. The smell of the damp, muddy earth and the sight of pink cyclamens peeking through the rocks were an integral part of my childhood.

I mustn't forget the magnificent beaches of the Mediterranean, its salty waters, the scent of the clear ocean air, and the "song of the sea:" the sound of the waves crashing against the shore. The cries of watermelon peddlers walking up and down the beach now brings on a surge of nostalgia.

Our shared adventures ended when the Bzostek family moved to the United States, where Moishe passed away several years later. Shoshana died in Israel in 2007 following a prolonged illness. Their eldest daughter, Zvia, returned as well, serving in the army and settling there, where she lives today with her husband Amos and their three children. Zvia's younger sister, Dalia, still makes her home in the United States with her three daughters and her grandchildren. We have stayed very close and keep in touch regularly.

* * *

Following the Yom Kippur War in 1973, my parents sold their home in Neve Monosson and moved to Rehovot, while my grandmother Babbe moved to Yahud to be near her sister. When she fell ill, my parents took care of her with love and devotion. She returned to live with them for a few more years, until she was unable to recognize the people around her. As home care became impossible, Grandma moved to a nursing home, and a few years later passed away.

My eldest brother, Yehuda, was born in October 1958, and I came into this world in September 1960. Raffi was born in January 1968. Although the three of us all grew up in Neve Monosson, Yossi, my parents' youngest son, was born in July 1977 in Rehovot, where my parents still live. We have all raised our own families and have led typical lives: weddings, funerals, ups and downs. My father retired, but unable to sit at home and live the "easy life," took a full-time job as a truck driver for an El Al subsidiary. He thought that this job would be calm compared to what he had done in the army and as a manager.

Everything was to change dramatically and unexpectedly the day of the accident.

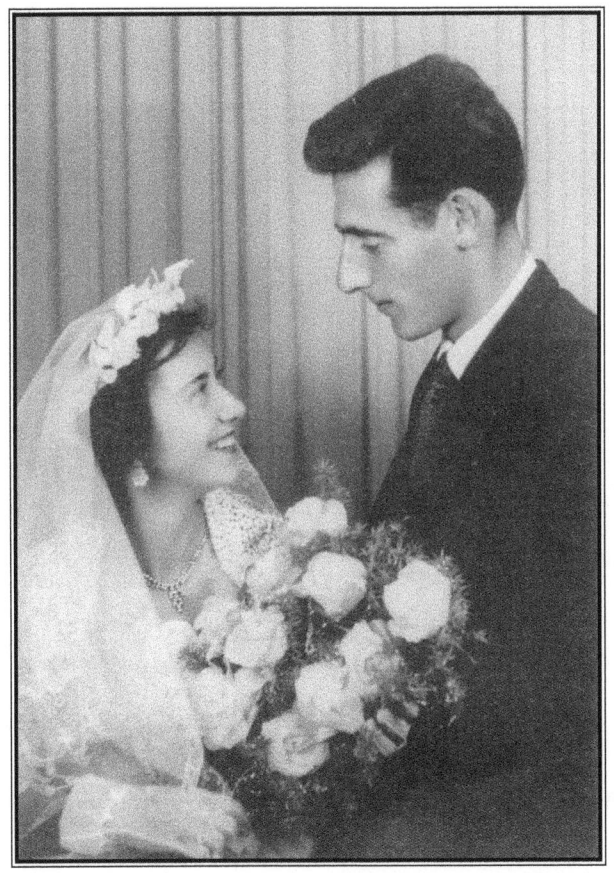

Wedding day: November 5, 1957

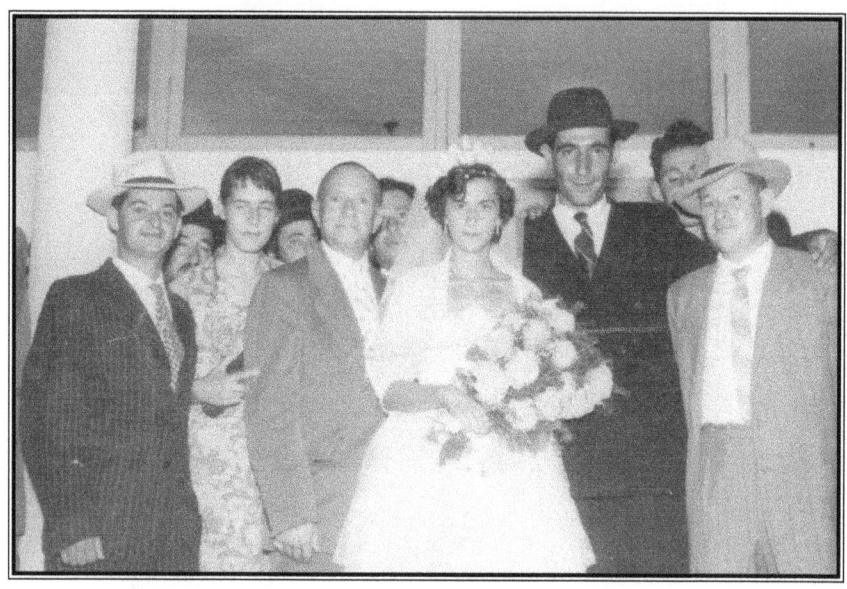

**My parents, Frida and Meir.
Efraim (Fred) Monoson is standing to the left of my mother.**

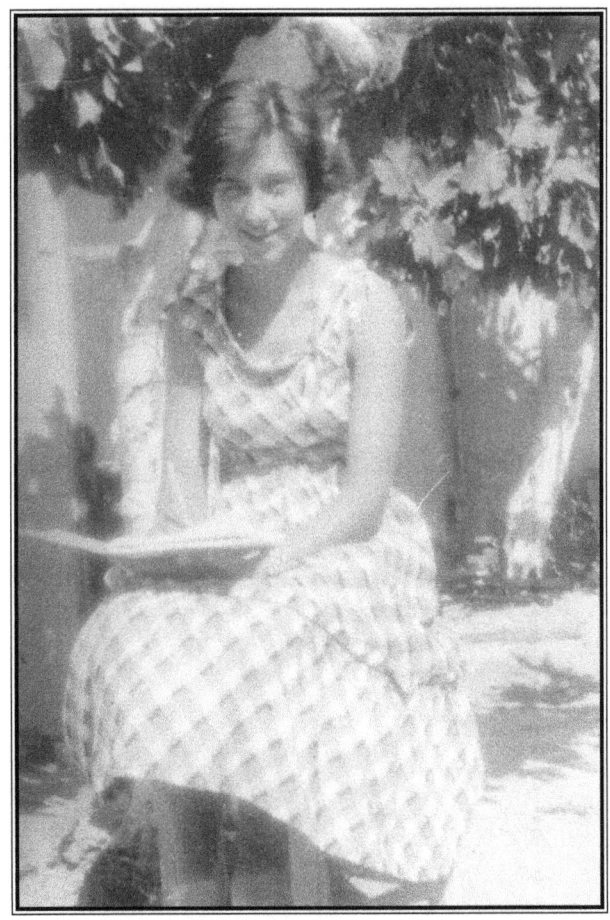

My beautiful mom in the Kibbutz.

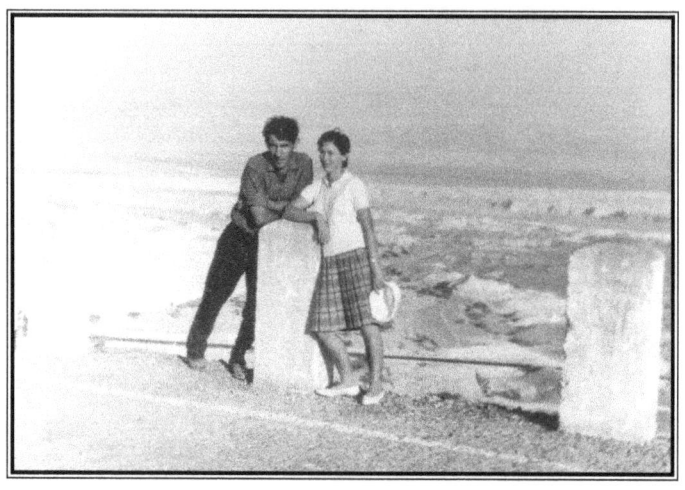

Mom and Dad enjoying an outing.

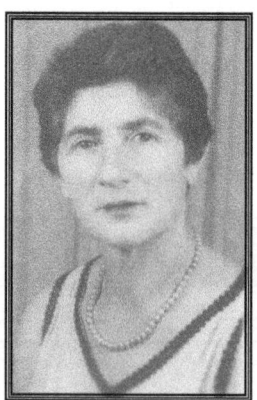

Our beloved grandmother, *Babbe*,
the late Zina Surik.

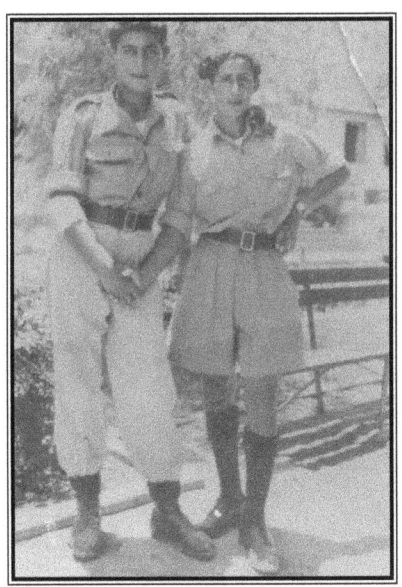

My dad with the late Chiam Feldshtein on their first day in the army, only two days after my dad arrived in Israel.

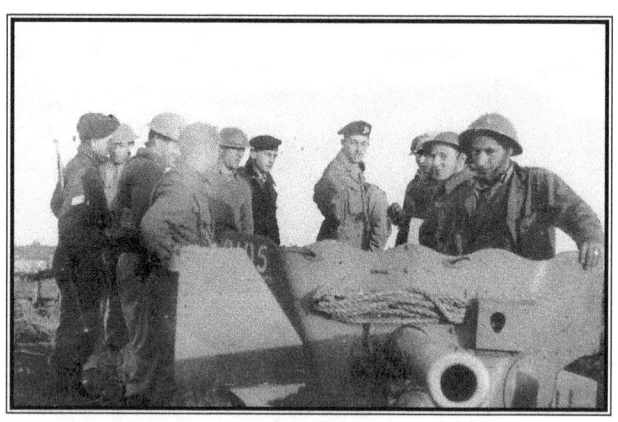

**Dad, on the far-right,
in a tank training exercise.**

The Will To Live

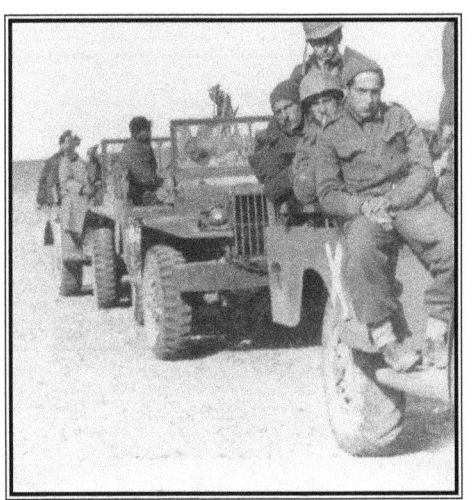

**On the way to capture Eilat.
Dad is at the right of the photo.**

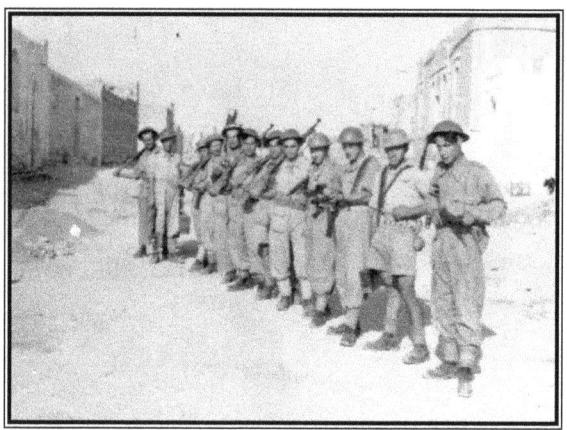

**One day after the occupation of Ber-Sheva.
Dad is again at the far-right.**

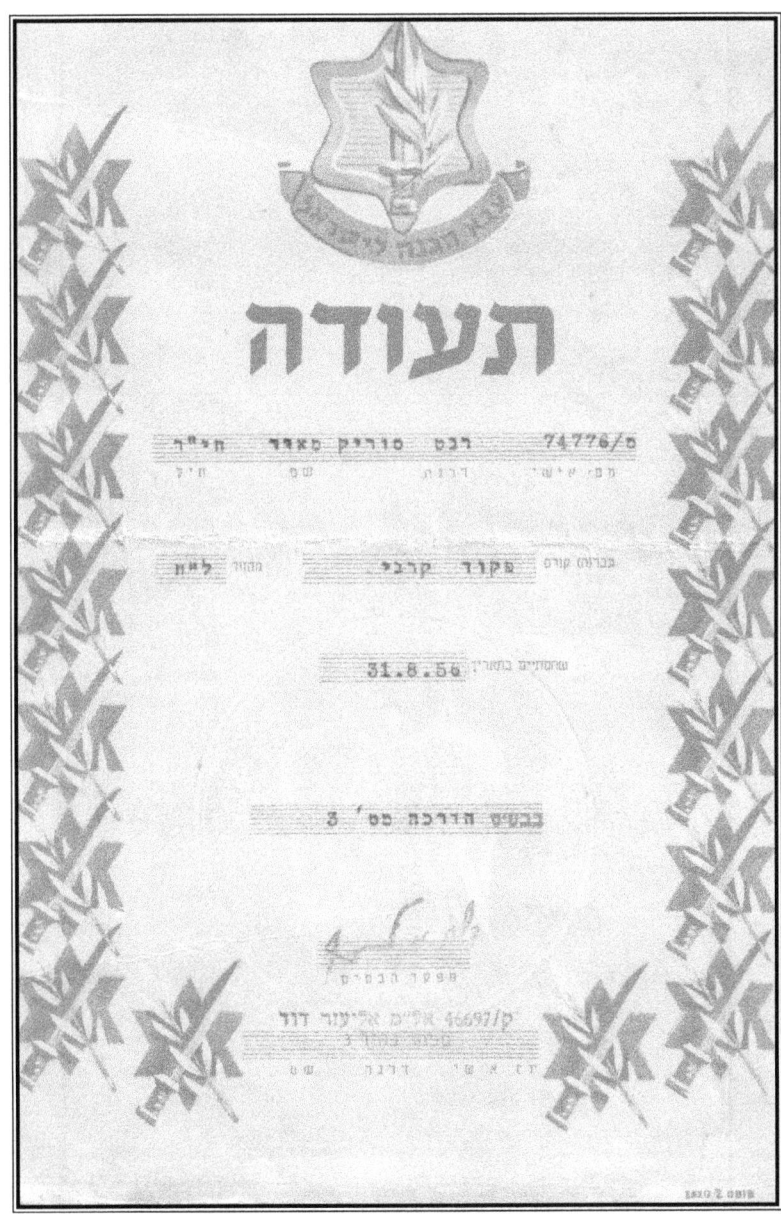

Dad's trainer's certificate signed by David Elazar, the future commander in chief of the IDF.

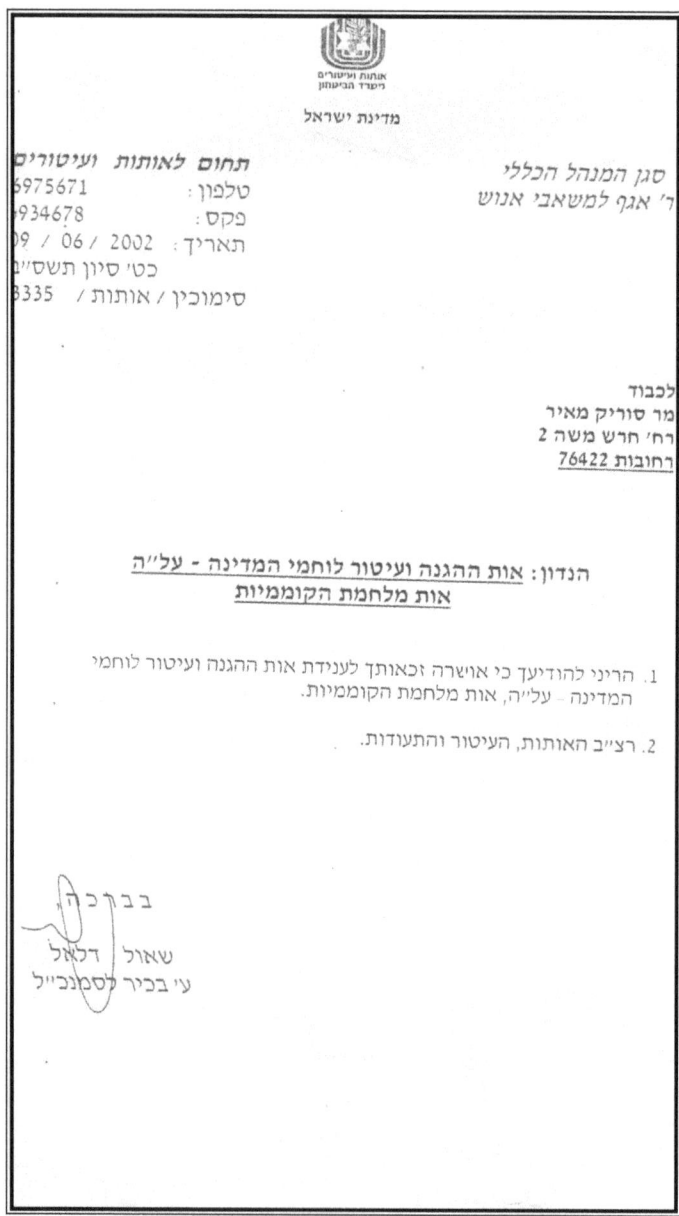

An award given to my dad for his service in the War of Independence.

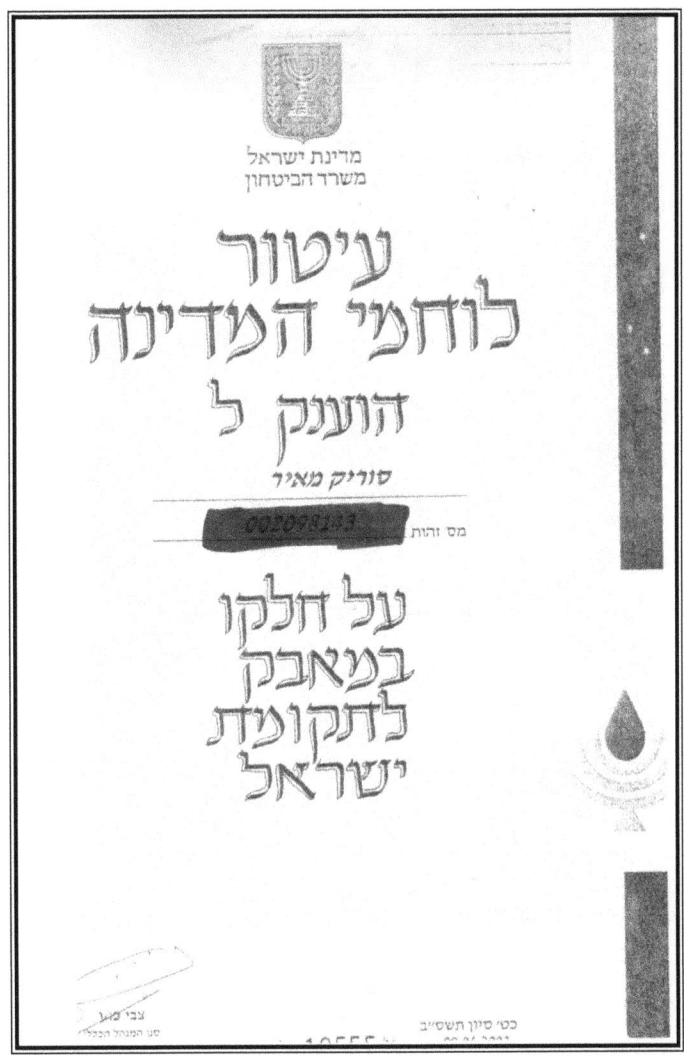

Another of my father's service awards.

Chapter 1
The Accident

It was August 9, 2000, 8:30 p.m. A critical event was taking place at the Kfar Shmaryahu intersection that has all but become routine in Israel: yet another car accident.

For me, however, this accident was very different. Despite not being present, I can still hear the sound of screeching brakes and the deafening sirens of ambulances, fire engines, and police cars. This time, it wasn't just another item on the evening news. This time it was my father, *my father*, who was in the truck. It was he who was injured.

The rescue teams worked tirelessly. After sawing the front of the truck in two, they were able to get my father out. His fate was decided in those very moments.

"What's your name?" asked a male voice.

"Meir," replied Dad faintly.

"He's alive, he's alive," whispered the emergency serviceman.

"Meir, what's your family name?"

"Surik. My leg hurts. I can't move my leg."

"Don't worry, Meir, we're transferring you to the hospital, and they'll take care of your leg there," replied the paramedic softly and sympathetically.

"Where do you live, Meir?"

"In Rehovot, 2 Moshe Harash Street."

"What's your home telephone number?" the doctor asked; attempting to assess Dad's awareness while distracting his mind from the pain.

Dad mumbled his number without hesitation.

Accompanied by loud sirens, the ride to the Ichilov hospital in Tel Aviv was the beginning of Dad's battle for life. It was to be a long, grueling fight.

* * *

"Hello?" said my mother as she answered the phone.

"Mrs. Surik?"

"Yes, speaking," replied my mother, hesitantly.

"I'm calling from the emergency room at the Ichilov hospital," said the voice at the other end of the line.

"What happened?" asked Mom anxiously.

"Is Meir Surik your husband?"

"Yes, what's the matter?" Mom asked impatiently.

"Your husband has been involved in a car accident. We're taking care of him. You'd better come to the hospital."

My mother froze.

"Raffi, Daddy's been in a car accident," she yelled towards my brother.

He ran to the phone but was able to obtain only a few vague details. All they knew was that Dad was alive. That was all that mattered. He was alive.

With heavy hearts, Mom and Raffi called the rest of the family in Israel and left for the hospital immediately. The news hit hard, shocking the entire family. Everyone's thoughts were racing: "What if they didn't tell us the whole truth? What if he's no longer alive and they didn't want to give us the bad news over the phone?"

The unknown was hard to bear.

Everyone was distressed and confused. How could Dad have been involved in a car accident? He was cautious on the road, known for his slow, careful driving. How could this have happened?

Yehuda, my eldest brother, and Yossi, the youngest, made their way to the hospital too. They received an update en route. Only I, the lone child living overseas in Canada, was unaware of the drama taking place.

After Mom and Raffi arrived at the emergency room, Raffi was the first to see Dad. He was fully conscious, but looked dreadful: his head was big and swollen, the size of a watermelon. Though he was awake, he was quite dazed. His face betrayed the pain he was experiencing.

The doctors were too busy to give the family any detailed information, and were able to share only their preliminary findings:

"We don't have a clear picture of the nature and scope of the injury just yet, but it's clearly serious and complex. We also know that several internal organs have been damaged."

The area surrounding Dad's bed was completely chaotic. The medical team prepared to move him to the operating room (OR) to perform what they referred to as "emergency surgery."

Before Mom was able to utter a word, Dad was transferred to the OR. She was left stunned and silent, not having had the chance to say goodbye.

Chapter 2
The News

It was 8:30 p.m. in Montreal when I answered the phone. I was surprised to hear my eldest brother Yehuda's voice on the other end of the line. I froze. Without calculating the time difference I knew it was the middle of the night in Israel, and Yehuda, who didn't call very often, would never have phoned at such a late hour if it hadn't been an emergency.

"How are you, Nechama?"

His voice was ominous. There was no doubt in my mind that something terrible had happened. Words cannot describe how I felt at that moment.

"What's wrong, Yehuda? Why are you calling so late at night?"

"Dad was injured in a car accident driving his work truck. I didn't want to call you, but I have no choice."

A wave of faintness came over me, filtering through my entire body. I trembled, afraid to ask how badly Dad was hurt. Yehuda, who understood exactly what

I wanted to know, answered the question that was never asked.

"Look, Nechama, I don't know very much either at this point. All I know is that Dad's been badly injured, and that he's on his way to the OR. His condition has been classified as critical."

"Who can I call for some details? When will I get more information?"

"I have no idea. I don't even know what kind of surgery he's going into. I think it involves his leg, but I'm not sure how long it will take. I'll call you in an hour."

My brother hung up. I was like a statue; motionless, with the telephone still in my hand. The only sound in the room came from the receiver dial-tone. I was disconnected from my family, powerless to be involved, unable to help them during this terrible crisis.

I called out to Shiri, my daughter, who was sixteen at the time. She was in her room with a friend who had planned to sleep over. Due to the circumstances their arrangement was cancelled, no unnecessary questions asked.

"Mom, I'm sure everything will be okay," Shiri said, attempting to soothe me with her soft, sweet voice.

I didn't cry. At times like this I usually become quiet and restrained. The people who know me best know that it is a calm that cries out to the heavens.

After attempting to console me, Shiri broke down. My daughter has had a raggedy pillow since she was about a year old. Before she falls asleep, while she watches TV, or when she wants to have some private time, she takes the pillow and strokes it on a certain side, in a certain spot, at a certain angle. At this difficult time the pillow was a refuge and a source of solace, absorbing the ocean of her tears. Michal, my eldest daughter, who returned home at 10:00 p.m., received the news with reserved silence. Just like me, she sat in the living room, stunned. For a long while she didn't say a word.

After the initial shock, we tried to think of what we could do so that I could fly to Israel as quickly as possible. It was late; travel agencies and airline companies were closed for the day, but I managed to find the home telephone number of an agent I knew and arranged to meet her at her home at 8:00 the following morning.

I still had not heard a word from the hospital. I was happy not to have any news.

Chapter 3
Traveling to Israel

I was standing at the entrance to my travel agent's home at exactly 8:00 a.m. the next day.

Mary, an elderly woman who is a Christian Arab, was raised in Jaffa and had immigrated to Canada many years before. She speaks perfect Hebrew with a strong Arab accent. Despite poor health, she made every effort to keep on working.

"Why bother with all the hassle?" I once asked Mary.

"Honey, I have to keep busy. Once in a while I even make a few Liras (dollars) to send to my family. I have a brother in Israel who's very sick, and I have to help out. Besides, I meet nice people," she replied warmly.

I had been buying my airline tickets to Israel through Mary for years. She was reliable, honest, and offered exceptionally personal service. However, that morning, despite her best efforts, she was unable to find an available seat on the flights leaving the same day.

"Mary, I must leave for Israel *this morning*. I don't care what airline I fly or how much the ticket costs. I'm leaving for Israel today, even if I have to stow away as cargo!"

"Listen Nechama," Mary said, "we must go to a travel agency downtown and find you a flight. I'll take you to the wholesaler that provides all the travel agents with their tickets, and I'm sure we'll find a seat on a plane today. This can't be dealt with from home, with no computer, making endless phone calls."

"I'm ready. Let's go," I said quickly. I was comforted that my good-hearted friend was, as always, ready to help.

Mary used her influence on the employees of the travel agency, and her efforts bore fruit; she managed to find a seat on a flight leaving for Israel via Toronto that day. In order to make my flight to Toronto, and then the connection to Tel Aviv, I'd have to be at the airport within the hour. How would I manage to prepare in just sixty minutes? I thought of the swift maneuvers I'd seen in films, and went into action. As Mary worked on confirming my seat and issuing the plane ticket, I called Michal.

"Michalooshe, I need your help, quickly."

"Whatever you need, Mom."

"I'm about to take a taxi and head home. Get my passport from the big bag in the bedroom. Throw whatever you think I might need into a carry-on bag. The taxi driver will wait and then take me to the airport. I have one hour to get there."

"I'll get everything ready right away, Mom."

A few minutes later I was sitting in a taxi, breathless, explaining to the driver what we were about to do, and trying to assess whether he had what it took to get me to my destination on time. Fortunately, he was a young, spunky driver who was thrilled to be given the opportunity to exceed the speed limit in order to please his customer.

"You just make sure there are no cops around," he said half-jokingly.

Michal waited for me in front of the house holding my passport and a carry-on bag she had filled with a few essential items. I said goodbye quickly, without going in or changing my clothes. I promised her I'd call from Toronto with the details of my connecting flight. I didn't even have a chance to say goodbye to Shiri. Michal let everyone in Israel know that I was on my way, and they were relieved to hear the news.

The taxi driver proved to be multitalented during our ride to the airport, exhibiting speed, familiarity with the roads, and – most importantly – patience and tolerance in the face of the honking and cursing he endured from furious drivers due to his crazy antics. He was relentless, and thanks to him my mission was accomplished; we arrived at the airport moments before the gate closed. Air Canada flies to Toronto every hour, but if I had missed this particular flight, I would have missed my connection to Israel.

Check-in was quick, as I had no luggage. I boarded the plane with the carry-on bag Michal had packed for me. I found my seat and dropped into it, winded. I took a deep breath. As the plane took off, my thoughts kept racing. I had no idea what had transpired during the morning hours or how I would find my father. The connecting flight to Tel Aviv was the longest I'd ever experienced, every minute feeling like an hour. Time seemed to stretch on forever. The tension was unbearable.

The flight arrived at Ben Gurion airport on Friday the next day at 7:00 a.m. Raffi was waiting for me, his eyes red. He told me that Dad was still in critical condition. We got into his car, not wanting to waste a single minute. An hour later we arrived at the gate of the hospital in Tel Aviv. I was trembling with fear. The path leading from the parking lot seemed endless; I felt as though we were going on a nightmarish ride down a long, dark tunnel winding on to infinity. The moment I'd reunite with the rest of my family was the light at the end of the tunnel.

Chapter 4
Reality Check

Life had come to a full stop from the moment of the accident until that Friday.

Despite the early morning hour, the whole family was at the hospital. Everyone breathed a sigh of relief as soon as I appeared in the Respiratory Intensive Care Unit (ICU) waiting room.

I received an update on Dad's condition. It was still considered critical. He was taken to the OR due to severe fractures in his legs that required immediate surgery. He also had multiple fractures on both sides of the pelvis, as well as fractured ribs, which were damaging his lungs. He suffered respiratory distress because of this and was connected to a respirator. Fortunately, he had no head injuries; but his general condition and vital signs were extremely unstable, and he had already received two blood transfusions. We were then told that he had been removed from the OR before surgery could be performed, because he would not have survived the operation. The physician assured us that when and if his condition allowed, he would be taken back to surgery.

At this point, I had not yet seen my father. Entry into the ICU is very restricted in terms of the people allowed in and the times during which they are permitted to enter: only the immediate family members can visit, in pairs, for fifteen minutes at a time, assuming that there are no extraordinary events taking place. Urgent, unexpected incidents are quite common in the ICU. All we could do was to remain strong and united, relying on the skilled medical team to do everything they could. Our only wish was for Dad to live. If that hope was realized, we knew we'd be able to handle whatever challenges arose in the future.

And then, finally, the moment I had been waiting for arrived. Two family members were permitted to enter for a fifteen-minute visit. Mom walked in with me after introducing the team with whom she had spent the last forty-eight hours. We were led to a large, air-conditioned, and well-lit room. There were eight beds in the room, four on each side. The room was at full occupancy, and each patient was connected to several machines.

"There's Dad," I said to my mother, as though she didn't know where he was.

The doctor gave me a few minutes alone with my father, and then returned to offer some explanations about his condition. Dad was covered with a white sheet, and his neck was supported by a red brace. A monitor hung above his bed displaying his vital-signs. There were machines on both sides monitoring the five different bags of fluids dripping into his veins. He looked good. He was asleep and seemed peaceful. The doctor explained that he was fully conscious but sedated. This was done not only to manage the pain but because it was a necessity as he was connected to a respirator.

The following days oscillated between hope and despair. Even the smallest update from a doctor determined whether it was a good day or bad. One thing was always clear: our dad was a real fighter. He'd fight to win … even the toughest of battles.

*　*　*

Each one of us dealt with the pain and fear of the situation differently, so we decided to share the necessary tasks according to our individual abilities. As I was a nurse, I naturally became the link between the medical team and my family. It made no sense for each of us to chase after the doctors with questions; if they had to respond to each family member separately, they'd be spending more time with them than with the patient. I made every effort to remain calm and collected so that I could offer my family strength.

Yehuda manifested his stress by not eating. For days he consumed only coffee and cigarettes. A *lot* of coffee and *many* cigarettes! He became an expert at knowing where all the coffee machines were located throughout the hospital and what the quality of the coffee was in each machine. For two whole weeks Yehuda was absent from his work and home, except for a few short trips he took to see his wife and children. He drove Mom everywhere and stayed with her at night as we didn't want her to be home alone. This task was of the utmost importance to us all.

Raffi was having difficulty coping with the chaos in the hospital. The traffic of doctors, nurses, social workers, and specialists in and out of the unit drove him mad. While each expressed their opinion on their respective fields of study, even visitors and relatives of other patients had advice and words of wisdom to offer. This combination of advice and opinion didn't necessarily contribute in a positive manner to the overall atmosphere, and so, from time to time, Raffi took it upon himself to relieve me at night when the hospital was quiet. He also undertook an important responsibility requiring much time and endless patience: dealing with the paperwork relating to the accident. When one is involved in a car crash or a work incident, the wheels of bureaucracy begin spinning. When one is the victim of a combined car and work accident as my father was, the family is faced with a real challenge. Treated with painful and insulting discourteousness, Raffi was given the runaround by each and every one of the institutions involved.

Yossi, the youngest of us all, maintained his optimism throughout, and rather enjoyed being involved in the medical aspects of my father's case. He quickly became my right-hand-man and took an interest in medical terminology, asking me about Dad's medications, their dosages and their side-effects. Sometimes he'd have questions for the medical team, and they were happy to offer whatever information they could. Yossi assisted me greatly each day, and his captivating and contagious smile was a constant source of comfort to our family and the hospital staff.

Mom had her own role. As we were all still spending our days in the waiting room of the ICU, she made sure we were all fed. Very well fed, being a typical Polish mother! Since Mom had great difficulty sleeping, she'd wake up in the middle of the night and prepare a huge variety of sandwiches, pasta, pastries, schnitzel and vegetables, burekas, hamburgers, nashes ("light" snacks), and copious amounts of coffee. These meals kept us going the whole time Dad was hospitalized.

Mom always tried to put on a brave face, making a show of strength and resilience, "so the kids don't break down," as she told a family member of another patient. "If the kids see me break down, it will be that much harder for them," though, truth be told, she occasionally gave in to her grief, crying once in a while. She kept saying all she wanted was for her

"Tzuptzik" (pronounced Choup-chick in English) not to suffer. That was her nickname for Dad.

Now, each of us had our mission. We knew what we had to do, and this gave us the confidence we needed to help Dad. We would be at his side in his struggle for life.

Chapter 5
The Conference Room

Ten days had passed, and Dad's condition continued to be critical. He was still connected to every imaginable machine, including the respirator. His blood pressure was extremely low and unstable, and the mercury in the thermometer didn't go below 40.5°C (104.9°F). It was impossible to tend to the severe fractures in his two legs, pelvis, or ribs due to the overall complexity of his injuries, the erratic function of his heart and lungs, and the various infections he was fighting.

On the morning of the tenth day, our family was called into the office of Dad's doctor. The initiative itself was alarming. Sitting in the waiting room of the Respiratory ICU for days on end taught us that when doctors have good news they hurry over to tell the family without holding meetings. The demeanor of the nurse who informed us of the doctor's request was also ominous. We gathered in the room around a large, round conference table with no conception of the magnitude of the bomb that was about to drop.

The doctor sat at the head of the table without any documents or medical files. He described the critical nature of Dad's condition, explaining that despite the treatment he'd been receiving, he had shown no signs of improvement and had not even stabilized. We knew Dad was in a critical state, but did not expect to hear the doctor's cold and harsh description.

He uttered his words with an air of indifference that shocked us.

"Look, given my update and the conditions I have just described, I believe the chances Meir will recover from his present state are very slim, maybe even unlikely. The problem is that even if we are to assume he will not remain in critical condition, what will his quality of life be? Even if he makes it, we are certain he will be completely handicapped. He will not be able to stand or walk, that's for sure, and he'll suffer from other complications as well."

There was dead silence. We felt helpless. Not saying a word, the doctor looked at us one by one, without averting his gaze, letting his words sink home. Then he broke the silence, asking:

"Is that what you wish for him? Do you think that's what *he'd* want?"

As soon as he uttered those words we all burst out crying. Needless to say, we were in no condition to consider the matter or to come to any conclusions. The doctor hadn't left much room for hope. What decision was he expecting us to reach?

We all left the doctor's office with our heads down, staring at the floor. The ICU head nurse was waiting outside and immediately called us into her office. Behind closed doors she told us that this particular doctor was known for his pessimistic approach and that one of his intentions was to avoid giving families false hopes. At the same time the nurse said we should be prepared for the worst. Whatever explanations she gave, we were all upset with the doctor – not for being direct, but for being so piercingly cold. Raffi was particularly angry.

"What an insensitive son of a bitch," he said. "I understand what he's trying to tell us, but why be so blunt at a time that's so difficult for us? Does he really think we'll give up? That we'll let Dad die? What an idiot."

Although I dared not ask my family, I had to ask myself the question the doctor had proposed: Was it worse to let Dad die, or to have him hang on and live a life he wanted no part of? Would he live a life of misery and dependence on others? What would be worse? Who were we to decide for him?

* * *

My work as a nurse means that I encounter many different aspects of the human condition. I often witness difficult, sad situations on a daily basis. I see people who have led full independent lives, and who, in a split-second, are reduced by a stroke to being a prisoner in their own body. One day a man is on his way to the bank, and the next he needs someone to push his wheelchair, feed him, change his diapers, and manage his finances. The pain and despair in these patients' eyes is heartbreaking. On the other hand, I also see people undergo traumas that leave them completely paralyzed, but despite everything, they continue to smile, enjoying the small, simple things in life that they had previously taken for granted.

The head nurse's words of encouragement offered us the hope we so needed during those moments. Not an illusion; just hope. The doctor, on the other hand, had embedded his formed opinion in his question, as though he was expecting our decision to correspond to his point of view.

I proceeded to have a tough internal dialogue, questioning myself, wrestling with my moral dilemma. Finally, I reached a verdict. In response to the most difficult and most important question – did we have the moral right to make decisions on Dad's behalf? – I reached the conclusion that we had no right to do so, as *all* the doctors had claimed he had no brain injury. Therefore, Dad had the ability and the full right to make his own choice. I knew that if he did not have the will to live, he wouldn't make it, and if he did, he'd stay with us. When I approached my mother and brothers with my feelings and these thoughts, I found we were all united. We love our father to the depths of our soul, and we knew we'd support and encourage him no matter what.

He would decide for himself.

Chapter 6
The Surgery

Two difficult days … Dad's temperature was still very high, and his overall condition was completely unstable. His right leg was rotting right before our eyes. His foot and ankle were blue, almost black. Even a non-medically trained person could tell there was no blood flowing to the area. It was a life-or-death situation.

It was August 22, almost two weeks since the accident, another day in the hospital. Raffi went home to Rehovot with Mom the night before so she wouldn't be alone. Yehuda had just returned to Tel Aviv, reporting for his 6:30 a.m. shift, having slept for only a short while after seeing his family in Haifa. We sat in the waiting room sipping the coffee he had brought from one of the machines he had come to know so well. I was reporting the events of the night, when suddenly one of the ICU doctors called us over. We jumped out of our seats.

"Your father's right leg is not doing well. We have to perform an amputation immediately in order to save his life. We did the best we could to avoid it, but there's no alternative. The necessary arrangements are being made to transfer him to the operating room as we speak."

"When will he be operated?" we asked.

"As soon as the OR is ready and we receive the blood units we requested in case we need them," replied the doctor.

"How long does this kind of surgery last?"

"Not long. About an hour and a half," replied the doctor courteously.

"We'll wait to hear from you."

The doctor waved goodbye and quickly made his way back to the ICU. Yehuda and I looked at each other, distressed but not surprised. We accepted the surgeon's pronouncement like devoted soldiers, without question or hesitation. During the preceding days, I had feared the doctors might not decide to amputate Dad's leg in time and that he'd die as a result. As it turned out, they were waiting until they believed the operation would succeed, until there was nothing left to lose. That time had arrived and I felt better after talking to the doctor. As he explained the procedure, his tone of voice had conveyed a sense of optimism. This was my only consolation.

Yehuda and I called Mom and the rest of the family to notify them of the surgery. They were all on their way to the hospital, just like every morning. That particular morning however, was not like any other.

The two of us sat outside the operating room, which was only a short distance from the ICU. Within a few moments we saw Dad being led down the hospital's narrow hallways, anesthetized, his body attached to every imaginable machine including the familiar respirator. The medical staff stopped as they went by, allowing us to kiss Dad before he went into the OR. Then the doors closed. The hospital hummed with activity, but we remained silent, anxious and apprehensive. Was that the last time we were ever to see our father? Despite our grave concern, we remained hopeful.

That morning, given that Dad was about to undergo emergency surgery to save his life, the doctors didn't ask for a consent form to be signed, sparing us the need for agonizing deliberations and tough decisions.

Up until that moment I thought that my flight to Israel had been the most difficult time of my life. I had no idea what awaited me once I arrived, and the anticipation had been terrible. However the next few hours waiting for my dad to leave the OR were even tougher.

Regardless of the doctor's assurance that the surgery would take about an hour and a half, Yehuda and I told the other family members that it was scheduled to take three to four hours. During the first days of Dad's hospitalization we had decided to tell each other the truth, even if it was difficult and painful, no matter what the circumstance. However, that day an inner voice told us that it would be best to lie. So we knowingly, intentionally, lied to our family, because we were sure that if the surgery would take longer than scheduled, everyone would be fearful. Further anxiety was not what we needed. It turned out to be a very wise decision on our part.

The hours we spent waiting for Dad to emerge from the OR caused Mom to reach her breaking point. Angry with herself for going home to sleep rather than staying with her husband, she was extremely frustrated and cried inconsolably, refusing to believe what was happening. She didn't want to think of the moment when Dad would open his eyes and discover he was missing a leg. Of course, Mom feared, as we all did, that this discovery would lead to an emotional crisis. But most of all we feared for his life, which was in danger more than ever before.

Yehuda and I sat close together near the OR entrance, holding tightly on to each other.

"There's still time, there's still time," we told the family, attempting to calm everyone down.

An hour passed. We had not received a word. Thirty more minutes passed. No one came in or out of the room. The ticking clock made us all tense and edgy. We felt every second go by. The doctor had promised that the operation would take an hour and a half, and there we were, ninety minutes from the moment the surgery began, having heard nothing; not a single word.

We knew it was not a good sign. We should have been told at least *something* by then, but the hospital staff wasn't providing any information. We continued sitting outside the OR in heavy, nerve-racked silence. My head was swimming with thoughts. The doctors had been very cautious when they had presented us with Dad's chances of recovery, promising nothing. "We hope he holds up," they said. We wondered if he would.

Two hours went by and we still hadn't heard anything. Yehuda and I were losing our minds. My whole body was shaking; I couldn't stand on my feet. Yehuda held me close, trying to soothe me, even though he couldn't hide his own feelings and nervousness. Raffi paced the hospital corridors worriedly, back and forth, round and round. The tension was unbearable, so intense that not one of us was able to console the other. Mom preferred to stay in the ICU waiting room, where she sat with Yossi in tense anticipation. She frequently walked over to us, eager for a report, although she knew that we'd inform her as soon as we received any news. Even so, every few minutes, someone – Raffi, Yossi, and of course Mom – would approach us wanting an update.

Yehuda and I went in and out of the OR secretary's office, desperately hoping to receive even the smallest tidbit of information. She repeatedly told us, with growing impatience, that as soon as she heard anything she would pass it on to us. No doctor or nurse had exited the operating room; none of us had any idea what was going on behind the closed doors. Three-and-a-half hours of unbearable tension went by, and then suddenly the OR door opened wide. The entire staff emerged, pushing and surrounding a bed with our father and Mom's beloved husband in it – alive. Dad had done it again.

The orthopedic doctor, who knew the family well, quickly smiled. His smile was warmer than the scorching sun on a hot Israeli summer day. That said it all.

"It's okay," he said, "we were even able to treat the left leg. That's why the surgery took so long. I'm sorry for the stress you had to go through, but the patient's well-being was most important. He survived the surgery, and we hope he will cope with all the complications it entails. We'll do everything we can. His condition is still critical, but it is now stable. We're transferring him back to the ICU, and we'll talk to you later."

Dad was lying in a bed, covered with white sheets, still under anesthetic. We couldn't see his missing right leg. We saw only what we wanted to see: our father, alive.

It was the first time since Dad had been hospitalized that we heard the word "stable." We all burst into tears, but this time they were tears of joy. The word that had just entered our official medical vocabulary – "stable" – received new meaning. Those six little letters could hold a world of hope.

Strangers shared our tears, each having their own tragedy or their own survival story. Everyone identified with us, becoming our extended family at this time of trouble. I sobbed and sobbed, the tears flowing from my eyes like water pouring from a faucet. However, when I cry, everyone else around me smiles; they know I only cry at good news.

* * *

The orthopedic doctor was grinning when he met us in the ICU waiting room several hours after the surgery. Only then did he have the time to explain to us why the surgery had taken so long. After amputating Dad's right leg and stabilizing his condition with several units of blood, the decision was made to take advantage of the situation and operate on his crushed left foot. We expressed our gratitude as the doctor humbly gestured "You're welcome."

Dad's vital signs began to improve. The problem disturbing us more than anything at this point was how he'd cope with the new reality forced upon him. I believe that the will to live overcomes all else in times of crisis; even the closest people are unaware of the unspoken physical and emotional powers their loved ones hold within. My father was going to live; now our family was about to begin coping with new challenges. Now we'd need those hidden powers.

Chapter 7
Friends, Family, and Faith

I have always believed that at times of crisis, those who are close come closer, and those who are distant fade away.

As they say: "A friend in need is a friend indeed."

Hardly any of our friends disappointed us; in fact, even people we expected little or nothing from visited and made telephone inquiries, providing much needed encouragement. Our entire extended family offered continuous support on a daily basis.

Some of our parents' neighbors, people with whom they exchanged only "Hello" and "Good morning!" arrived at the hospital, wanting to help. El Al flight attendants who had worked with Dad during the preceding years, and whom we had never met, made great efforts to come to the hospital. This gesture touched us deeply.

Two very special people will be etched on our hearts and memories forever thanks to their dedication, their never-ending concern, and their eternal love. The late Chaim Feldstein (Dad's friend from Europe) and

"Petia" Tzerbin (May he live a long and healthy life!) were particularly helpful and supportive during our family's crisis. At the time Dad was in the hospital, Chaim was also very sick; he had been suffering from larynx cancer for many years and had lost his voice as a result. With the aid of his beloved wife, Bruriya, he would call everyday to ask how Dad and the rest of us were doing. As he was unable to talk, he would write down what he had to say on a piece of paper, and Bruriya would convey his messages. After a while, Chaim and I developed a telephone communication code: when I asked a question, one tap on the table meant "Yes," two meant "No."

Chaim insisted on coming to Ichilov hospital to visit Dad, which meant he had to take public transportation from Haifa. The distance involved showed how important it was for him to be with Dad and us during those troubled times. Over the course of the first few days we tried explaining to him that his visits were unnecessary, as he would not be able to see Dad due to the restrictive entrance policy of the ICU. We asked him to save his strength for the days to come, but he dismissed our arguments. One day, he appeared early at the hospital with his wife, and as they sat with us in the waiting room, we communicated through the little notes he'd scribble. His penmanship was beautiful, but he would write in tiny, almost microscopic letters, as though trying to save paper. He had become accustomed to that method of communication as a result of his illness. Chaim had an extraordinary sense of humor, and he was always telling jokes and incorporating funny stories into our conversations. He even jotted down some short jokes for me on the little white pieces of paper he held in his hand.

Over the previous days, the doctors had hoped to perform a certain test but had refrained, fearing that any movement would cause a drastic deterioration in Dad's condition. During Chaim's visit, and thanks to the stability in Dad's vital signs, a decision was made to transfer him to the X-ray department. Though it was a small development, for us it was a mini-celebration.

Within a few minutes, a nurse and two support staff led Dad's bed and ventilation equipment through the waiting room and down the hallway. Chaim was beaming with joy, not only because he was sharing in the happiness we were experiencing but because he was able to see Dad, even for a brief moment, as he was led down the halls. I felt that this was no coincidence; that it had all happened that morning precisely because Chaim had been there. I told him what I was thinking, and tears began flowing from his eyes. We shared a long moment of silence, understood only to us.

Petia and Sima Tzerbin displayed extraordinary loyalty too. Despite their poor health, they called daily to receive updates on Dad's condition. Petia's promise to "pray for my brother" encouraged us and warmed our hearts.

These are the kinds of people Dad has as friends. They are our family.

Chapter 8
Recuperation

As the days passed, Dad began to recover. He started weaning off the medication that had been stabilizing his blood pressure. His antibiotic treatment had been completed, and the anesthesia was terminated. A dramatic process was now set in motion because Dad had not been unconscious, but rather drugged for the unbearable pain.

The process of awakening from continued anesthetization is a long and frustrating one. The patient wakes up gradually, and this makes it difficult to tell just how conscious they are. Additionally, in extended cases like my father's, the implications of prolonged medication are unclear. Dad had been anesthetized and ventilated for about a month. We anxiously awaited the moment when he'd regain his senses and recognize us. When he first opened his eyes, they remained open for over twenty-four hours, as though he was trying to catch up on the recent weeks.

Despite his steady gaze, there was nothing to indicate that Dad recognized us or was even aware of his surroundings. Besides that, he didn't close his eyes for a single second and, as a result, developed a severe eye infection. Yet another one! Forty-eight more hours passed, and I began noticing that the look on Dad's face became clearer, less fixed and distant. I also noticed obvious signs of pain and discomfort. I approached the head doctor, pleading with him to relieve my father's agony, even if that meant drugging him again. Dad's discomfort was our biggest fear. The doctors promised that they wouldn't let him suffer but decided to use painkillers rather than anesthetics because they wanted him to wake up. Their approach met with our approval and great relief. We felt that they were fully cooperative, and we valued their openness, empathy, and understanding of the issues that preoccupied us.

I was thrilled to see Dad open his eyes. I had feared that I would have to return to Canada before I'd see him that way, before he'd be able to know that I'd been there, by his side, twenty-four hours a day for a month. Thirty days had gone by since I'd left my family in Montreal. This also meant thirty days of absence from my workplace, taken without advance notice.

My original return date had been set for two weeks following my departure, but after the first ten days, I notified the airline that I would not be able to return at that time. The airline representative was courteous and understanding, and suggested that I call to reserve a seat when I was able to fly back. After a month, I was finally forced to make the painfully difficult decision: to extend my stay in Israel again or to return home and prepare for my next visit. I felt torn between two worlds. After considering the matter with my family in Israel and abroad, I decided to go home and to fly back as soon as Dad showed further signs of recovery. Only one family member disagreed with this decision: my younger brother Yossi. He was saddened by my impending departure, and not wanting me to leave, tried to convince me that I made the wrong decision.

My constant presence at the hospital and my calm and collected demeanor in times of crisis had made everyone stronger. That was the least I could have done.

Two days later I was on my way back to Canada.

Chapter 9
Faith and Religion

The little square indicating religion on my ID card says that I am Jewish. I am not Jewish by choice but because I was born to Jewish parents whose ID cards also say they're Jewish. Every person has a different kind of faith in his or her heart, and each person has a different name for it. One believes in God, another in human kindness. I was brought up on a set of beliefs devoid of hypocrisy, based on deeds derived from honesty, stemming from love for family and friends and a desire to assist those in need. That was the type of education my parents instilled in me where "religion" was concerned. There are those who keep the laws of *Kashrut*[4] and are considered religious, despite the fact that they do not honor the Ten Commandments. While my parents do not keep kosher or observe other Jewish traditions, they raised me to respect the "Golden Rule," which is the same in every culture: "Do unto others as you would have them do unto you." This teaching has always been the root of my spiritual foundation.

On the other hand, my father could surprise us all with his occasional "religious" devotion. In times of

---

[4] Kashrut means Kosher laws as they apply to diet and other everyday activities.

desperate need, people are sometimes willing to adopt customs and perform deeds that they would not ordinarily identify with in their everyday lives.

* * *

My father lay in his bed in the ICU, his eyes wide open. We were still unsure how aware he was of his surroundings or how sharp his senses were. One day, several smiling *yeshiva*[5] students appeared, holding large Torah scrolls. The hospital staff brushed them off by telling them that the nature of the unit prevented them from entering. The boys accepted this and were about to leave when something completely unexpected happened: my father motioned to the nurse to let them come in. The nurse, stunned by father's alertness and quick response, was deeply moved and decided to bend the rules. She quickly ran after the boys and brought them back to the room. They surrounded Dad's bed, and as they danced and sang holding the Torah scrolls, Father kissed the Torah, filled with emotion and pride. All of us – the family members, doctors and nurses – were dumbfounded by this surprising spectacle. We all had tears in our eyes.

During the coming days, as we attempted to decipher the mystery, we reached the conclusion that Dad wanted to cling to *something*. The *yeshiva* boys

---

[5] Yeshiva is a school for religious men.

appeared at the right time, in the right place; they were a symbol of faith, and steadfast devotion.

The following day, at 6:00 a.m., while the "divine spirit" still hovered over us, my uncle called me. I was surprised to hear the phone ring so early in the morning, but he said he had good news and that good news should not be put off. The previous day, his daughter had made a special trip to see a great, well-known rabbi in order to tell him about Dad's accident. She recounted the story of the event, the injuries and the overall situation, expecting to receive his blessing. The rabbi listened attentively and replied: "The decree will be overturned." The meaning of that affirmation was that Dad would recover.

My uncle, who was fully aware of Dad's position on such manifestations of religion (which I share), attempted to substantiate the rabbi's credibility by telling me that a few weeks prior, my cousin had visited the same rabbi regarding another man who was gravely ill. To her dismay, the rabbi was evasive, and refused to grant his blessing. As she left the rabbi's home, she called to inquire about the man's condition and was told he had passed away moments earlier.

My uncle was extremely emotional. He believed that the rabbi knew exactly when he could or couldn't offer his blessing. At that moment, I also wanted to believe, to cling to anything that would provide us with positive reinforcement. Now, looking back, I know it was not religion that gave me hope for my father's recovery, but the faith and will planted deep in my soul which defies labeling.

* * *

I tend to perceive religion, and many of its leaders, as exceedingly primitive. As a case in point, the crossing of the Red Sea in the story of the Israelites' exodus from Egypt is very difficult for me to grasp. How could it be possible that the sea parted and the Jews were all able to pass through on dry land, unscathed?

I cannot comprehend the idea that there is an entity sitting up in the sky, watching us, aware of our every action, each and every moment of every day. Does this God condemn the hypocrites who manifest their faith once a year at Yom Kippur but ignore His commandments the rest of the year? This is ostensibly irrelevant as, of course, God loves us and will forgive us for anything.

Religious people believe that when bad things happen it is God's will. Even if an honest person goes bankrupt, a young innocent child dies, or an unexpected factor enters our life and ruins us, we still have to believe that *God still loves us* and that we must accept our lot. One day we will presumably understand the reasons behind our misfortunes.

One of my closest friends is religious, and although we have differences in beliefs, I love and respect her dearly. She does her very best to follow all Jewish laws, and one of the most important aspects of Judaism is celebrating the Shabbat from Friday sunset to Saturday sundown. Religious Jews, including my friend, operate no mechanical machinery throughout that time. One Shabbat eve, she made her way to her synagogue on foot, as she does every week. The synagogue is about a twenty-minute, fast-paced walk from her home (no harm in that; walking is good for one's health). When the prayers concluded, she made her way home in the pouring rain, arriving soaked to the bone because it is strictly forbidden to open an umbrella during that time. My friend tried to explain to me, with enviable inner peace and serenity, that her walk in the rain was a pleasant one. It even felt sublime, she said, as it was done out of absolute respect and love of God.

I still have trouble accepting this explanation, particularly since the following day I had to fulfill the edict of calling on the sick, as that same friend had contracted pneumonia.

I much prefer my parents' version of "religion."

Chapter 10
Remote-Control Care

Back in Canada, I returned to a normal routine, or at least as normal as possible considering the circumstances. I went back to work at the hospital and resumed cooking and cleaning at home. When Dad's condition was stable I received regular calls three times a day, but if something was even a little out of the ordinary, I was notified immediately, day or night.

I used to call directly to the ICU to receive "live updates." The fact that I now knew the people I was talking with on the other end of the line gave me a sense of trust and comfort. The staff was very kind and patient and answered all my questions with courtesy.

After almost a week at home, I had a day when I needed those immediate "live updates." Dad was undergoing another very difficult surgery, this time on his left foot. During the course of the operation he had to receive a few more units of blood, making a grand total of twenty that had been transfused since the accident. My family was upset and in a nerve-racked, anxious state, as the long hours of waiting for Dad to come out of the OR had taken a severe toll. Meanwhile, I was worried sick at home waiting for a call.

At last the phone rang, and on the other end of the line I heard my little brother say: "I am waiting for you to cry." That meant good news! In fact, the operation had gone so well that everyone was hoping that Dad's blood pressure and respiratory status would finally be brought under control. Once that happened, it would be possible to consider transferring him from the ICU to a regular unit. Of course, on hearing the new development, I broke down in happiness, as was expected.

* * *

In Canada, and across the seas in Israel, the whole family now knew that when Dad regained consciousness and became aware of how we had all fought for his life, he would also realize just how much love surrounded him. In the little battles, as well as the big ones, our care and his will had triumphed. We felt that this pride in himself and his family would also give him the strength to win the next round in his rehabilitation. My mom began gathering her energy for this moment so that she would be able to offer him all the hope and encouragement he needed to mend his shattered body.

However, my father was not yet out of the woods in regards to his basic physical condition. His low blood pressure was still posing a problem, as it was one of the most significant side effects of both the pain-control medications and the anesthetics. Additionally, Dad's body temperature had been slightly above normal prior to this surgery, and it now began to inch up to its former levels. Both Mom and Yehuda stayed at the hospital overnight, although entry to the ICU was totally forbidden during those hours. I tried to convince them that it was more important that they get some rest, but they insisted on staying. I understood, because most probably I would have wanted to stay if I'd have been there. There was no need for further convincing.

The effort I made the following morning to speak with the chief doctor was unsuccessful. I was left very disappointed and frustrated because it was a Friday, and I knew that he would not be there during the weekend. I was anxious to know if he thought that there was any indication of a change in my dad's level of alertness.

Hypothetically speaking, my life in Canada had some semblance of normalcy, but the reality was that my entire world revolved all around Dad and my family. My thoughts and my heart were some place far across the ocean. Since I needed to be able to make contact at any time and from any place, I used to carry a few long-distance phone cards: one in my wallet, one in my bag, and another always in my pocket. Our conversations sometimes lasted just a few minutes and at other times more than an hour. There was always someone from the family available to talk with me around the clock.

It was then that I started to keep a journal. It came to be a vital part of my life. My writing not only helped me to focus, it served an important goal: to tell my father of all the events which had taken place during the past few weeks, especially the feelings we had been sharing. This helped me believe that Dad would hang on and stay alive. I was writing my journal for him so he couldn't go anywhere without reading his story. He needed to read those lines ... I depended on it.

Another day went by, then another weekend. I held a long conference call with my three brothers. They told me that one of the hospital's social workers had requested a family representative for a group-support discussion. She had begun initiating these group meetings as a family-therapy tool and had met with great success. Since each family had to deal with a different variety of issues, everyone could share their experiences and learn to deal more effectively with their own situation. When people hear that they are not alone, they tend to open their hearts and share their emotions.

Although the request was to have one representative from each family, it was no surprise that three Suriks had attended the meeting; my mom and two of my brothers. They left the session very happy because several participants were kind enough to take the opportunity to express their thanks for the support and encouragement that my family had provided throughout their stay. After all, *my* family had the "most seniority" at the ICU!

One of these participants, a Bedouin from the south of Israel whose brother had survived a complicated liver transplant, declared with tears in his eyes that he considered our family as his own. It was nice to hear that my mom and brothers were able to reach out and help others, despite being so occupied and distracted by their own troubles.

Most of the patients that were at the ICU when Dad was admitted were already transferred to a regular unit, and some had even been discharged home. One young man had been admitted suffering from a tooth infection. Although it subsequently spread throughout his body and nearly killed him, he recovered quickly and was in the ICU only three days. Nevertheless, he and his relatives returned to visit my parents and brothers soon after he had been released. That gesture touched our hearts deeply.

Unfortunately, two people died while Dad was still fighting for his life. They have left the struggles and the turmoil of the ICU for the quietest place ever.

Chapter 11
My Girls

I was certainly not the only one coping with Dad's accident. My family in Canada was also dealing with the situation, each in their own way. My daughters Michal and Shiri were just as worried as I was about their grandfather and were also learning to face my countless fears and regrets. One night, when we were sitting in the living room and watching TV, my girls noticed that my eyes seemed glued to the screen but that I was actually just staring into space. I had not even realized what program was on and was immediately given a lecture by my two children:

"Mom, Grandfather will be alright. He will recover slowly and his broken leg will heal. He will be okay. He is not the first person in history to live with one leg," said Shiri.

Michal added: "As long as his head functions, everything will be fine."

They began reminding me of people we had known who had faced various disabilities yet continued to enjoy their lives. They were aware of the fact that I was filled with helplessness and guilt because I was unable to stay in Israel to help my family and my father.

"Don't worry Mom, Grandfather will know that he is in our hearts and that we are thinking about him and praying for his recovery."

The words of wisdom and encouragement that my daughters expressed were the source of my greatest pride, and they were the ones to give me the strength I needed to cope with our tragedy. They said everything that needed to be said, and they said it all at the right times. Like me, they lived from news to news and, like me, they used to jump at every phone call from Israel.

Michal and Shiri love my parents with their whole hearts and are very attached to them. They always say that they are the greatest grandparents in the world, and both my children adore the affection and devotion that they demonstrate to one another. The girls also admire their grandparents' warm open-door policy, which they have had all their lives.

At the time of the accident, my daughters were both high-school students. Since then, Michal has completed her Bachelor's in business management at Concordia University in Montreal and has moved back to Israel. She currently holds a full-time job as an international relations manager, which requires many trips abroad.

She is also a full-time student at the Hebrew University of Jerusalem and is in the process of completing her Master's in communication and journalism.

Shiri has obtained her Bachelor's degree in social work at McGill University in Montreal (with great distinction!) and is currently working full-time. She plans to acquire more working experience before tackling her Master's degree. My girls are leading very busy lives but are never too busy to think about their grandparents. They call them as often as possible just to say "I LOVE YOU," and of course visit them every opportunity they get. For my parents, the relationship they share with Michal and Shiri is one which brightens their lives immeasurably. For my daughters, my mom and dad are the ideal grandparents, loving role-models who enrich their entire world.

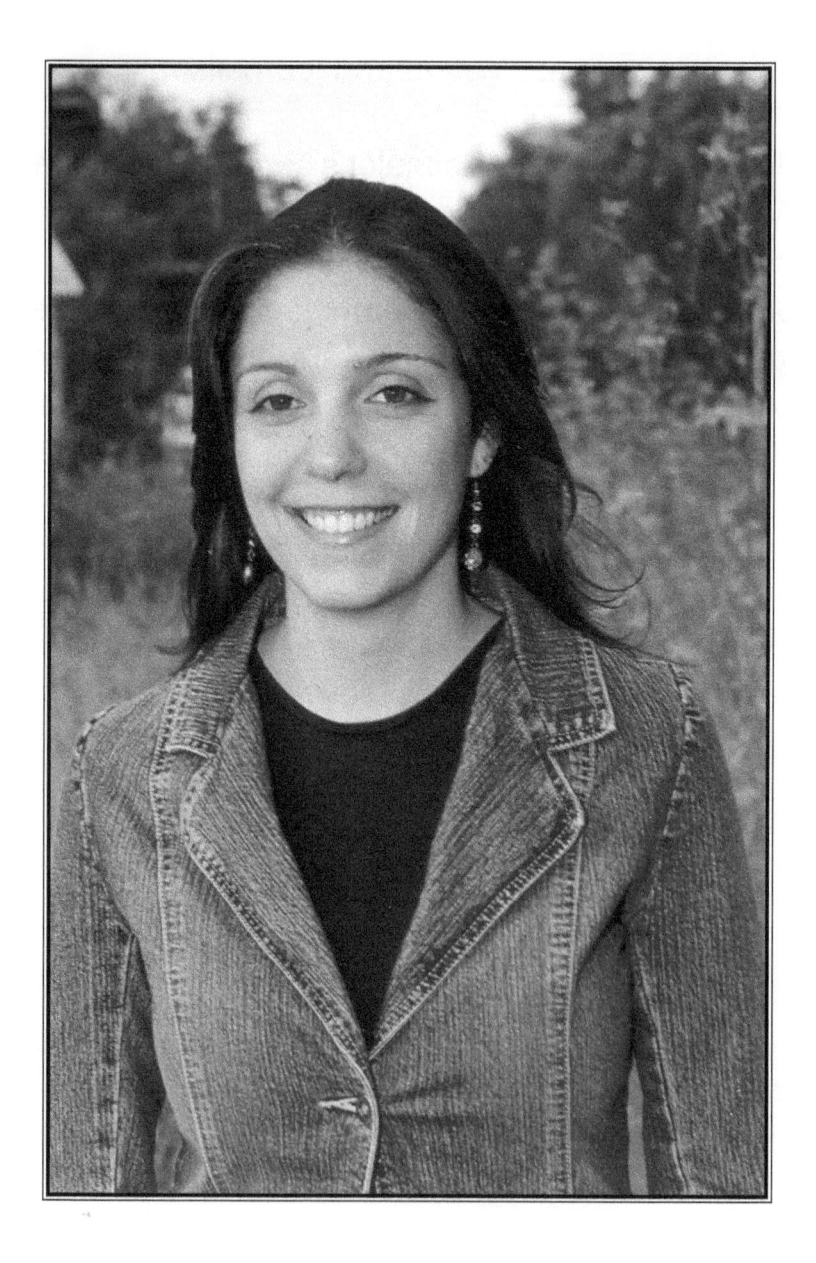

Michal Rosenbaum

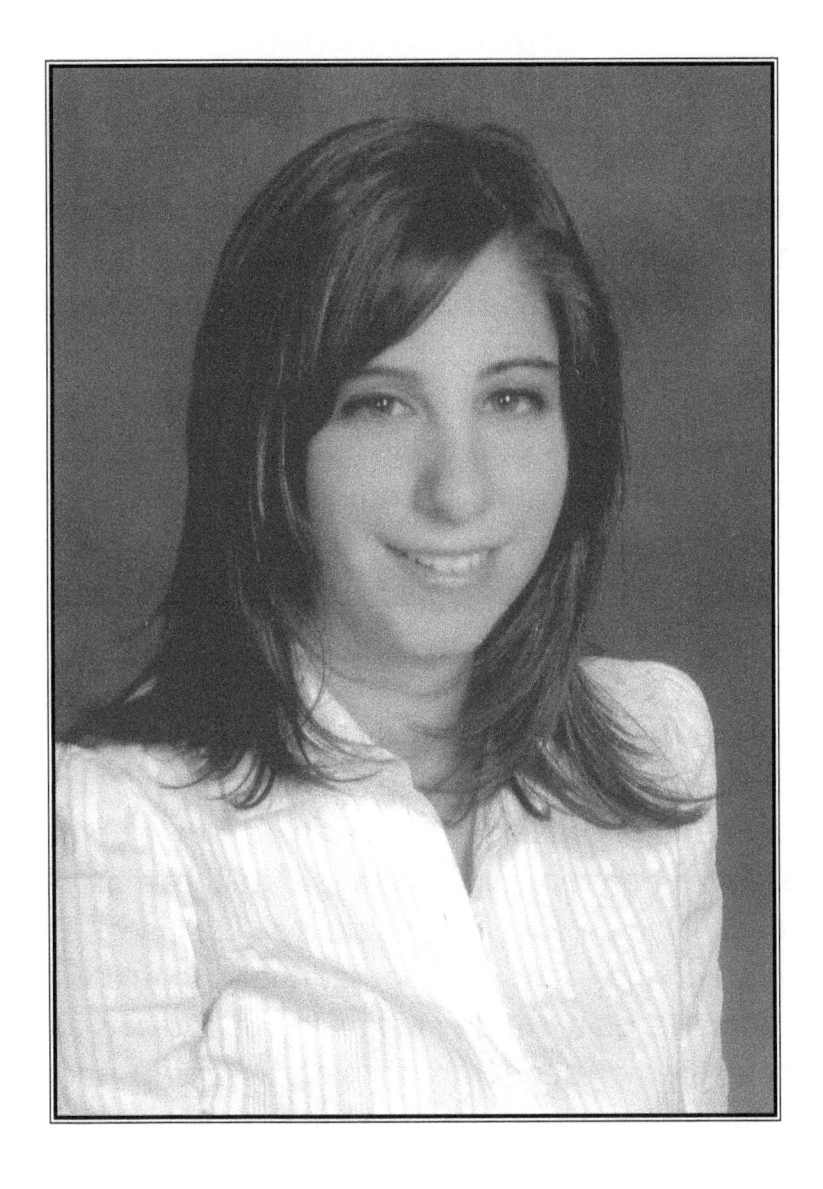

Shiri Rosenbaum

Chapter 12
Significant Smile

Another bad day passed by. Dad's fever continued to climb and we didn't know why. Additionally, his blood pressure dropped, and his respiratory distress became more acute as he received morphine for pain control. Morphine wasn't the best choice for Dad, but oh boy, it could have been a great help for the rest of us on that day. We certainly needed something to get our blood pressure down, as our anxiety and tension levels were sky-high. The situation could put any sane person out of their mind.

I had been waiting impatiently to speak with the chief doctor because I had an idea that I wanted him to take under serious consideration. I wanted him to consider the use of an epidural, rather than the morphine, to ease Dad's pain. The same epidural is given to woman during labor, so I figured that it would act as an effective pain-suppressant without causing either hypotension or serious respiratory distress. Another significant benefit of the epidural is that it would not cause any delays in neurological recovery. Of course, these were only my thoughts and suggestions; I didn't know what the experts were going to say or what kind of "action plan" they had in mind.

As hours passed, and after numerous attempts to reach the doctor, I got very impatient. I was about to pull my hair out. After being glued to the phone for so long and getting nothing but busy signals or answering machine messages that tell you "your call is important to us, thank you for your patience," my nerves were shot, and I was climbing the walls out of frustration.

Finally I had to go to work for my night shift. As I got to work, and after receiving the report from the evening-shift nurse, I tried to call the hospital again. Then a miracle occurred: the doctor himself answered the phone. I expressed my concerns about Dad's deterioration and, in a very diplomatic way, asked him about the possibility of treating the pain with an epidural rather than with morphine. He admitted that he hadn't thought of that option, but said that it would only be considered when the fever would fall to a normal range. I appreciated the doctor's honesty, as well as the fact that he was listening carefully to what I had to say. He provided me with the reassurance that I desperately needed, and this alone made me feel stronger and more secure.

At the same time I started to ask myself: "What am I doing here at work trying to solve other people's problems when I am not able to resolve my own? I reminded myself that my patients needed me, and that they needed my full attention as much as I expected the nurses at my father's hospital to be totally focused on him. As a health care professional I had to put my clients and their families first. As a human being, I felt the same responsibility.

I love my job. I love taking care of people and always give the best of myself, but since Dad was in the hospital, I felt that I had difficulties concentrating on my duties. I was just so worried that I was often busy calling my family whenever I had a free moment. That would happen regularly on every shift.

* * *

The thought that occupied my mind the most was how Dad would react when he became aware of what had happened. How would he deal with the realization that he was missing his right leg? That he could no longer dance or even walk normally. His leg was gone! How would he feel when he realized that he was alive only because he was connected to all these machines? He was attached to so much equipment by so many tubes. What would happen when he eventually figured out that he needed help for every single movement that he wanted to make?

Those questions wouldn't allow me peace of mind for even a moment, day or night. Was it possible that Dad would blame us? Should we have agreed to let him get to that state in the first place? Instead, should we have let him die?

The Will To Live

We all wished that when Dad would finally open his eyes, discover his total dependence, and realize that his life had completely changed, he would still not give up or lose hope. He would once again prove to everyone that he was tougher then ever, that his mental strength would overcome his physical disabilities, and that this inner strength would be the foundation and motivation for his will to live a long life beside his beloved wife.

It was 7:00 a.m. in Montreal, and I was just about to complete a night shift, when my little brother Yossi called me, sounding down. He told me that everybody was discouraged and frustrated after their daily visit, as Dad had indeed opened his eyes but had not shown any signs of expression. It seemed to them as if he were in a different place and in a different world. He didn't recognize his family and didn't react to his surroundings at all.

I drove home fast because I wanted to speak with my dad's doctor before he went home. This was the doctor that knew my dad's history from the first day of the injury. I got lucky and was able to reach him just as he was at the door on the way out.

In a very calm and peaceful way he showed interest in Canadian weather. He then asked about my health. I was about to explode because I really only wanted to ask him how my father was doing.

"May I ask you how my dad is today?" I interrupted gently.

He started laughing, and told me that he was happy to finally have encouraging news.

"Your dad's condition is improving day by day. At a certain stage I thought that we would need to start dialysis treatment as his kidney function was not good. Now it's off the agenda because there is a huge and unexplained improvement, and the kidneys are almost functioning normally."

He continued: "The level of consciousness has been improving dramatically as well, and that's a very important indication of positive progress in his general condition. I am very pleased."

I told the doctor how worried, concerned, and anxious my family and I were, as we were not aware of these changes. Nobody had told us anything. He kept explaining to me that my father didn't react to his wife and sons because he was "drugged out," and not for any other reason. Neurologically, there were no problems detected, and it was only a matter of time until he would start responding. He also added that Dad's breathing had improved so much that they were thinking about discontinuing the use of the respirator. These tidings were fabulous and I finally had excellent news to tell my family.

At the same time I was hearing this, Mom and Yehuda were at the ICU waiting room expecting my call, as they knew that I was about to talk with the doctor. It had often happened that I would call the doctor as my family was at Dad's bedside. We would talk, and then I would phone one of my brothers to report what the doctor had just said, all while he was standing right next to them.

Yehuda answered the phone and was thrilled when he heard me crying. He knew I only allow myself to cry when I am happy, so he started jumping for joy even before hearing what I had to say. I told my mom and Yehuda all the developments in detail, and while I was doing this, the glad tidings went through the cell phone to the rest of the family. The ICU sounded and looked a bit like a "news room."

However, after I spoke to them I realized that everyone but Yehuda had received the news with a kind of restraint. Their happiness was reserved because they couldn't see or feel the clinical improvement in the reality that the physician was describing. From what they had seen, there was no change.

Yossi then called me with many questions, and I didn't have the answer for most of them. He reminded me that I always say that we do not need to ask everything. Often, we can see the changes without being "medical professionals." If a certain medication is being stopped or reduced; if there is no fever; if the vital signs are stable, we know there has been an improvement. We can't run after the doctor for every little thing.

Yossi then asked how come we hadn't seen any of these significant clinical changes. It was difficult to answer. "We need to have patience, we have to wait and see," I told my little brother.

"I am so discouraged, Nechama. It's like receiving your pay slip, but the money isn't in the bank."

"Patience my brother, you must have patience. We know now that we are on the right track."

The miracle happened just a few hours after my conversation with Yossi.

Mom got to my father's room, and suddenly, he grabbed her hand and smiled at her.

Dad had awakened to life, and with him, so had my mom.

Chapter 13
Additional Worries

Dad was awake, and although we had been waiting so long for this, I felt troubled and distressed.

I was suffering because I was far away, and now it killed me that I was not at his bedside when he had finally shown real signs of consciousness.

I was bothered by the thought that my dad might wonder why I was not with him. He was not able to speak at that time, but it was possible that he was able to recognize his surroundings and see that his only daughter wasn't there. The thought that my father might think that I neglected him drove me out of my mind; I couldn't bear it. After all, how would he have known that, for the longest time, as he was ventilated and under anesthesia, I was next to him day and night? Every minute that I was beside him I would massage his hands and legs for as long as I had strength. I was determined to try and reduce the edema, the swelling and accumulation of fluids, to allow a better blood flow. In the same manner, I exercised his muscles with ROM (Range Of Motion) techniques to reduce muscle atrophy as much as possible. When the doctors and staff saw how hard I worked, they didn't say a word about visiting hours. Even at the times that they were treating other patients, they allowed me to stay in the ICU. They were amazed by both my physical ability and my will power to do everything I could to reduce the risk of other possible complications. Back in Canada, I hoped that Dad had felt my presence at those times and would remember that I was with him.

* * *

The real coping started the moment Dad awoke. We knew that he would need help around the clock and that pain management would soon become the most significant matter we had to face. He had made it this far, but now, in his condition, further pain could lead to death. When a person is suffering, they don't care about anything else, and certainly not about rehabilitation. Pain management is a serious matter because it leads to loss of appetite, insomnia, lack of social interest, and in general, decreased motivation. With these factors in play, patients often become immobile. This may result in the formation of bed sores and systemic infections. The most serious complication can be a condition called sepsis. Sepsis occurs when bacteria from a skin infection enter the bloodstream and spread throughout the body. This is a life-threatening condition that can cause death, and my dad was at high risk for all these factors. However, the most terrifying issue Dad had to face was the enormous suffering.

This meant that we needed to push for an immediate intervention regarding pain management.

I was hoping that Dad would know how to make the best out of his situation and cheer up. I was waiting to hear that he had smiled again, just to know that it hadn't been our imagination. I wanted the family to see the same kind of conscious smile that he had given my mom the other day.

* * *

For a full month, Dad had been connected to every medical machine and device possible. He had a nasal tube feed inserted in his nostril, his neck had a hard support to avoid any head movement, and he had a hole in his throat from the tracheostomy done to alleviate his breathing problems. Besides these, all his medications were administered through artery intravenous infusion. Furthermore, a blood pressure machine was curled up on his hand, his finger was squeezed by a clip to measure the oxygen level in the blood, and there is no need to indicate where the Foley catheter tube was coming from! All you could see were wires and tubes extending from every part of his body.

Behind the bed there were a few beeping control screens that reminded the casual observer of an airport control room. However, the patients in the ICU didn't look like your typical backpacking travelers. Many of them appeared as though they were on a completely different journey, maybe their last trip.

Not my father of course! I knew that he would recover.

Although the machines, the tubes, the wires and the beeps all caused us a certain inescapable anxiety, they were not the only factors worrying the family. While we admired the staff for their professionalism and dedicated work, we had to use a certain code to figure out what they were saying when they talked to us. For example, the doctors seemed to follow a policy of communication that embraced a very "restrained" method of information sharing.

It took us time to understand that this policy only served one purpose: to protect their own asses! They had devoted lots of their time, money, and emotions to studying, and they would not say even the smallest thing that might risk their reputations or raise issues of credibility. When a doctor gives you good news, you know that you can party, because if he had even the slightest doubt, he would not tell you anything.

So that day, when the doctor declared that there was a significant improvement in my dad's condition, it was a good reason for me to cry my eyes out.

The very same day, Mom, Yehuda, Raffi, and Yossi told me that Dad had without doubt recognized them. One look at his face said it all.

All of a sudden my family became a new species of "medical detectives;" analyzing every breath, every hand movement, and every blink of an eye. Each motion was immediately granted a new meaning:

"That was a call for help!" "No, he wants to drink." "What are you talking about? He is in pain. ..."

The Surik interpretation crew then tried to analyze the movement of his right hand: "He is waving good-bye." "He wants us to leave." "He wants us to get closer!" "He wants us to be quiet!" "He wants us to turn off the light?"

While everybody was so busy trying to figure out "what he wanted," Dad fell sound asleep.

Chapter 14
Between Desperation and Hope

The coming few days saw the family float between desperation and hope. After they had initially believed that my father had responded to them, Yehuda and Mom were now convinced that Dad had no connection to reality. He was staring into space and didn't react to conversation or physical contact. At the end of her regular daily visit, my mom broke into tears. She claimed that Dad had opened his eyes but was still deeply asleep. Everybody sounded depressed and discouraged, and it was especially heartbreaking to see my mother like this.

She is the true hero of this story, and all the way through she had tried to hang on to her hopes and keep her spirits up. Now, seeing her beloved husband with his eyes open, but without showing the slightest sign of recognition, was just too much for her to take.

After I got the daily report, I insisted on speaking again with the chief doctor, as if that would change my dad's condition. I knew that he didn't have a magic formula to wake Dad up from his deep sleep, but I was desperately trying to make sense of things; I just needed *something* to hold on to.

As I spoke with the doctor, he didn't show any signs of concern. His tone of voice was very calm, and he didn't reveal anything that would have demolished the hope we had. He repeated that he was not worried and that it was only a matter of time until Dad would respond. He was surprised to hear that my family was so worried, and he was particularly troubled to hear about my mom breaking down. He liked her, and talked all the time about how brave and devoted she was. He couldn't understand why my family reacted the way they did, so I explained to him:

"Well, nobody talks with my mom or my brothers. They don't like to disturb you, and so they rely on *you* to provide the information. I often have difficulties in reaching you by phone, and they are just hanging on thin air until they get the news from me."

When he heard this and found out about my mom's mental state, the doctor jumped. He apologized for the miscommunication and for the insensitivity of the whole unit for not informing the family about the positive changes. He explained, with lots of patience and compassion, that there was no way that Dad's head could clear up like magic, especially after such a prolonged use of high dosages of narcotics.

I thanked him dearly, but then sat back and thought things over, concluding: "How much power doctors have!" Truly, a few words of explanation from a doctor can change everything. All they need to do is to think about what the family is going through and how much they rely on their expertise. What comes out of a doctor's mouth can let a family dream peacefully or leave them spending a sleepless night full of worries.

The next morning we were filled with joy to discover that the doctor was right. The neck support had been removed during the night, after holding Dad's head for a whole month. We were amazed to find that even the respirator had been disconnected. We all followed his every breath with apprehension, hoping he would manage. We were all biting our nails observing these new developments. Every lungful Dad took in; we did so too, as if we could give him some extra oxygen.

Chapter 15
Pessimism

Dad was still treated with high dosages of morphine.

Our family was torn between the approach of keeping Dad "pain free," and of gradually discontinuing the narcotics so that he could slowly regain consciousness. We wanted to be sure that his brain was still functioning, and I always believed that as long that there was no brain damage we could overcome all the other problems that might arise. We needed a sign that the doctors were right, and we were starting to get impatient.

Yehuda was very irritated and worried. He refused to believe the doctors that there were clear indications of a big improvement and just didn't want to hear anything about it. He always had the tendency to hang on to a negative perspective, and in my father's case, he was so afraid of disappointments that he chose to adopt a permanently pessimistic attitude. I tried to talk him into seeing the light at the end of the tunnel by pointing out the big changes that had taken place over the past month, but it was like talking to a wall. I had to leave him to deal with the situation in his own way.

Dad's fever went down to 38°C (100.4°F). We didn't observe any neurological changes, but the doctor expressed satisfaction on the way his badly injured leg and hips were healing. All of a sudden, just as the doctor was listing the significant improvements and describing how pleased he was with the general progress, my father went into serious respiratory distress. The oxygen level in the blood went down to 80 percent. A big commotion started around his bed, and before we knew it, he was connected to the respirator again via the tracheostomy. Yehuda immediately came out with one of his pessimistic declarations: "The more expectations you have, the more disappointed you'll be." He reminded us cynically of what he used to say over and over again whenever there was an improvement: "Don't get into a state of euphoria...." We couldn't argue with my brother now.

He sounded angry, but was only worried to death like the rest of us.

Despite everything, I felt quite positive about my father's recovery. We had failed to disconnect him from the respirator, but it was a medical impossibility to do this in one shot anyway. In almost every case it is a weaning process which can take weeks or even months. Unfortunately this was just another example of a failure in communication between doctors and families. Only after this first attempt to discontinue respirator support did the doctors explain to my family that there was no need to panic: "It takes time until he'll be able to breath on his own. It will be like that on and off until we will be able to wean him off the machine."

If this explanation had been given to my family before the intervention and not after, they would have understood and nobody would have gotten "hysterical." It definitely set Yehuda so far back in his faith in the medical profession that he lost total trust in the doctors' opinions.

My brother Raffi has a real temper. When the doctor said: "What's the panic about?" he couldn't control his emotions. He turned and walked out quickly, stomping so hard you could hear his anger from a distance. Suddenly, out of nowhere, he hit the wall really hard with his fist. Everybody around was furious, and figured that it would be better not to talk with him just then. Unfortunately, as his hand was swelling rapidly, Yossi had to accompany him to the emergency room. This time, I was happy not to be around! After a few hours wait at the ER, Raffi started to lose his patience so Yossi scolded him: "You better keep your left hand safe!" At that, they both burst into uncontrollable laughter and were finally able to relax.

When they came back, Raffi's hand was all bundled up with a heavy dressing. Of course, he had fractures! When Yehuda slapped his shoulder as usual and asked: "So how are you?" Raffi said: "Oh, much better now ... I had been waiting to do that for a long time."

Meanwhile, back in Canada, I was in a tense situation. My family and I were about to move to a new house. A very difficult process to go through at the best of times, at this point it felt like the very worst time to be contemplating such a change.

It's hard to describe how complex everything seemed to be. My thoughts weren't into relocating, but I didn't have a choice, as the new lease had been signed previous to my father's accident. I comforted myself by thinking that after this transition I would be ready for my next trip to Israel.

I was far away, but so close with all my heart and my soul ... and so edgy that I was unable to sleep.

At night, just when I was about to close my eyes, I would see my dad's face in front of me, just as I left him at the ER. I would dream about him opening his eyes and smiling to everyone. I would see him joking, asking for food, and would hear him call for my mom to be always at his side. I could also see her suffer through my dad's pain and then I'd feel like my heart was torn apart. Minute by minute, hour by hour, it was all I could think about.

Chapter 16
One Month Later

On September 8 I was to celebrate my fortieth birthday. In July, not long before my father's accident, I received my parents' birthday gift by mail. It was strange that they had sent it so much earlier. It was as though they felt that something was going to happen, something that would prevent them from congratulating me on time. It was an important "changing 0" birthday, but the early present just didn't feel right.

When I questioned my parents about the early delivery and asked if they had forgotten my actual date of birth, they just told me: "You know Nechamale, that's an important birthday and we do not trust the mail. We'd rather your gift arrives two months earlier than one day later." These were their exact words.

Upon opening the parcel, I found a very special and emotional present: the most beautiful wooden square box, adorned with gorgeous, artistic, handmade engravings. Inside the box I found a CD with my picture printed on it. When I turned on my stereo and started playing the disc, I heard a beautiful song. Its lyrics and music were written about me and especially for me by my parents and my three brothers.

Everyone had done this together as a family project and had then taken it to a recording studio to be sung by a professional singer.

I listened to this CD with its one song over and over. I was filled with pride for this wonderful gift from my beloved and extraordinary family.

Now, after the accident, my only birthday wish was that my Dad would recover, that I would hear his voice on the phone, and that he would tell me, as he always did:

"Nechamale, that's it! I have a headache from your talking. We'd better finish before I need a Tylenol." That's how long my regular phone conversations with both Mom and Dad would last.

At this time, even though I wanted to speak to my family with all my heart, I was frightened of the phone, as long-distance calls often meant troubling news about Dad's health.

* * *

At 6:30 a.m. Montreal time, on my fortieth birthday, we all jumped out of bed to an alarming telephone ring. A cold sweat covered my forehead, and shivers traveled all through my body. I was frightened, because the day before a serious gall bladder problem had arisen. It had turned out that an invasive procedure was necessary, and so a drainage tube had been inserted. Now, the next day, we thought the call meant that complications had set in.

My brother Yossi was on the phone. The first thing he said was: "It's time to cry." He knew that hearing the early phone call can bring on a heart attack, and he didn't need the trouble of me being at the ICU.

He was excited and told me in one breath that, for the first time since admission, Dad had been transferred from his bed to a chair. Nobody had expected something like this to happen. At that time we were mentally and subconsciously trained to think only: "Life or Death."

My mother had been called to come in as usual, like every other morning. However, she never expected to see her husband sitting in a chair with his eyes wide open.

She was thrilled, and in a second, filled with energy for the days to come.

Dad was seated in a big, very fancy, leather La-Z-Boy. He was looking around and even turning his head, but his eyes still seemed distant and expressionless.

Mom was as happy as a woman that had just given birth. She didn't move from his side and was very busy with the simple acts that now became so significant. In the small hospital cupboard she had long kept a big shiny red bag with little yellow butterflies on it. Inside were Dad's shaver, smelly soaps, and aftershave. She couldn't wait to open that bag! That day, my fortieth birthday, she was busy from morning to night; shaving him, cutting his hair, and, so very gently, washing and creaming Dad's hands and face. Every time she touched him and looked at him, she was making love with her heart. She knew then, that very soon, Dad would be back.

As Yossi completed his breathless update, and as we were about to hang up, Yehuda came on the phone. I wasn't even given the chance to tell him that I had already heard the news.

Of course, I was just exploding with joy and happiness to hear my pessimistic bother giving me the same report, all in one breath, exactly like Yossi.

"Yehuda, today is the day for you to cry too," I told him. For once, he listened to his younger sister. Sure enough, seconds later, Raffi was on the line, excited and happy like there was no tomorrow.

I couldn't talk with Mom because she was too busy pampering her Tzuptzik.

Happiness filled my heart, but as the day went by, I began to be disturbed by the fact that Dad hadn't shown any signs of reaction to his new surroundings. We had been waiting a long time for even the slightest change, and now I was becoming frustrated and restless. I even started to have doubts about what the future had to hold for us, and mostly for Mom and Dad.

After a few hours in the chair, Dad was transferred back to bed with a mechanical lift. He looked comfortable and didn't show any signs of respiratory distress or discomfort. Yehuda then decided to take a drive home to the north to see his family. He missed them terribly as he hadn't seen them for many long days. As he approached his doorstep, even before entering his house, his cell phone rang. Mom was on the phone totally terrified. She told Yehuda that there was a big tumult around Dad, as his facial expressions showed signs of severe pain of an unknown source. All visitors including my mom were asked to leave the ICU while the doctors tried to figure out what was happening. Yehuda kissed his wife and two kids at the door of his house and then, like a madman, drove back late through the night to Tel Aviv. Fortunately, Raffi and Yossi were still at the hospital when the incident occurred.

The doctors and staff dragged in an ultrasound machine, and they worked hard to find the source of Dad's pain. Finally, they discovered that the gall bladder drainage tube had been displaced, probably during the transfer from the chair to the bed.

Very quickly the problem was solved, and as Yehuda arrived, our father appeared to be pain free.

My family was exhausted, but happy enough to call and sing for me:

"Happy Birthday."

Chapter 17
My Grandma

At the time of the accident, my mom's mother lived in a nursing home in Tel Aviv. This was a home that was divided into different units depending on the level of assistance needed. Our BabaLuba was an exceptionally alert woman with a very sharp mind. She was involved in all the social activities at the nursing home and was able to walk with a walker on her own. Because of these factors, she had an independent unit with a private bathroom, which came with a little kitchenette and a fridge. The only help she required was for her daily morning shower.

She loved to go to the main dining room for all her meals, not only because of the delicious food, but because of the room's elegant look. It had large shiny chandeliers, beautiful furniture, and sparkling, well-polished cutlery. The tables were covered with nice, well-ironed tablecloths and always set with fresh flowers. However, the highlight of the meal came in her conversations and interactions with other residents and staff. Especially the men!

My BabaLuba was extremely social throughout her life. Much as she cared about the look of the place she was living in, her physical appearance was no less important. On her own, she used to schedule her weekly hair appointment, which she kept religiously. Also, she was never caught "off guard" without her red lipstick on. Every evening after supper she had her regular company for a two-hour card game. She had a great sense of humor and always had jokes to tell, so these games were very popular with the other residents. Whenever there was a pause in the conversation, she would fill the awkward moment easily and gracefully, making up a joke or a funny story in the wink of an eye.

Mom and Dad used to visit her regularly every Friday afternoon, bringing the foods that she loved. Dad also used to help out with the little things she needed. When the accident occurred, she knew that he had been hospitalized but didn't have a clue as to how severe his injuries were. Nobody had had the courage to tell her that he was in a life-threatening condition, and we just kept putting off the moment of truth, trying to protect her. Every day she cried on the phone begging us to take her to see her son-in-law, and every day we had to find a different excuse to get out of it. She missed both my parents and their Friday visits, and she naturally became unhappy and worried, as she was a very smart woman. Mom then didn't have a choice, so she took a few hours off her "shift" at the hospital to go and face our BabaLuba with the news. My grandma broke into pieces when she saw her daughter. As my mother told her the story, she couldn't get over the gravity of the situation. She was so used to seeing my father active: driving, shopping, and doing everything for everybody, that it was impossible for her to imagine him without his leg, being so unresponsive. Mom did her best to comfort BabaLuba, and helped her realize that there were lots of positive changes compared to his initial prognosis.

Even after this talk, Mom still insisted that it was too early to take BabaLuba for a visit, and although we disagreed with her, we respected her decision and request. My brothers did their best to visit their grandmother as often as possible to cheer her up, and I called her regularly from Canada.

However, despite all our best efforts, the happiness that had always shone from her eyes and face was gone, as was her store of funny jokes and stories.

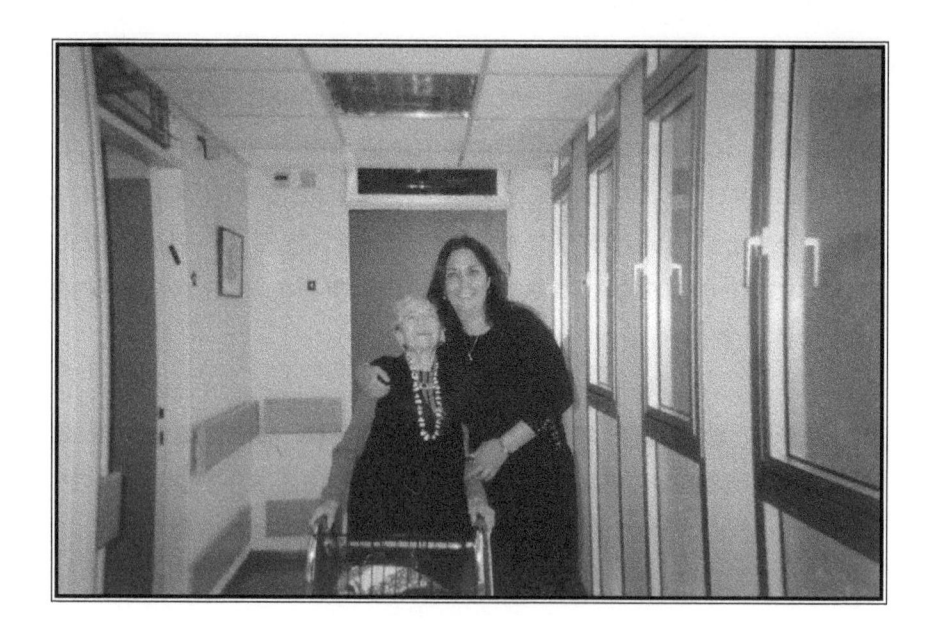

Nechama and the late Baba Luba, 2004.

Chapter 18
The Transfer

As Dad started to eat, his condition continued to improve. Although he wasn't talking yet, he looked more alert and his face started to regain its color. The gall bladder drainage tube had been removed, and most importantly he had gradually started breathing on his own. He was now transferred to sit on the La-Z-Boy "manager's chair" for a few hours each day. This appeared to be very comfortable for him, as he could sleep in it in the reclined position and thus tolerate it for longer hours. It was very important to have him in a sitting position, particularly for his lungs.

On the other hand, my family got more stressed out. While Dad was eating and drinking and often breathing on his own, he didn't talk at all, and it didn't appear that he recognized the people around him.

I spoke with the doctor in charge and asked him if he thought that Dad knew that he had lost his right leg. He was amazed at my question and said that there was no doubt that he was aware of it. "How do you know?" I asked him.

He said that he himself told Dad and that, from time to time, he had also observed him lifting his blanket while seated, looking at his stump. Again, I was surprised. All the staff knew that we were worried about Dad's reaction, but nobody bothered to tell us that the doctor actually spoke with him about his leg. That was a significant piece of information to forget! Although we didn't know how much my father could absorb, it would have made it easier for us to know that someone had talked to him. No one in my family had seen Dad looking under the blanket to check his amputated leg.

The doctor also told me that there was a huge improvement over the past few days in his kidney function, heart, lungs and neurological status. He expected that in just a short while, Dad would be transferred out of the ICU to a regular unit.

The doctor gave me all of this information only because I called him. Again, he didn't think about talking with my family sitting in the same room he was in. This information was important as it meant that Dad's life was out of danger. We had been waiting to hear this for so long.

I immediately called my family to report the news. They weren't too overwhelmed, and after they had listened, they concluded by saying an "AMEN."

* * *

The following morning at 6:00 a.m., a phone call got me jumping out of bed again. I knew that with every early long-distance ring there was a message. The situation was unclear, and like Yehuda, I had lost a bit of confidence and didn't know what to expect.

"Today is the best day ever, so cry already!" These were Yossi's words. Dad had been discharged from the ICU to the internal medicine unit. Everybody was very happy, but Mom was in complete shock. Although the move meant my father was getting better, the new unit was a mess and the conditions were poor. The room was very noisy and crowded, as it was being shared by six patients. My mom defined it as a "refugee camp." It was so hot that it felt like being in a sauna, and without air-conditioning, it was almost unbearable in the scorching Israeli summer. The smell of sweat was not easy to take either. Additionally, there was no doctor or nurse around to help when we had a question. It seemed that we had no-one to talk with, and Dad looked very restless.

However, only a few short hours later, it was amazing to see my dad start to communicate with my family using facial expressions and hand movements. He couldn't talk as the respirator was still on and off, but he was trying to say things that nobody could understand. His frustration about it was clear, and my mom was going crazy seeing him in that state.

I asked Yehuda to give Dad full and accurate explanations of his condition. He needed encouragement now and had to be assured that the respirator and his consequent inability to speak were temporary. We were worried that he thought he might be in that situation forever. I asked him to explain that Dad would eventually get a prosthesis and that everything would be okay. Most of all, I wanted him to tell Dad that although it was only a "hostel" compared to the five-star ICU, the ICU was for people whose lives were at risk, and that it was a happy sign that he had been moved out.

Yehuda thought that it was a great idea and enthusiastically took on the responsibility. Unfortunately Dad couldn't hear a single word, so the long explanation turned out to be a complete failure. In the ICU he had been treated with a type of antibiotic whose most common significant side effect was hearing loss. For some people this effect was permanent, but in most cases it was only temporary. For our family, however, it caused chaos.

We were all irritated and upset, but lucky that Yossi, our quiet, calm angel, was there to mellow everyone out. He sent Yehuda and Raffi out to take their "Ventolin" puff (smokes) and asked them to come back only after they both had a pack of cigarettes, a gallon of coffee, and at least a pound of smoked meat. Oh boy, were they happy to run away! In the meantime, Yossi went to the gift shop and bought a board and a box of chalk. He came back, and in a very relaxed way, sat with Mom on Dad's bedside and wrote to him, one sentence at a time:

"Your life is not in danger."

There was no response. They still didn't know what Dad could understand.

"You will be able to speak soon. The breathing machine is temporary." Now a big smile appeared on my dad's face. Mom and Yossi were thrilled! It was their first time seeing him react directly.

Yossi wrote: "Dad do you understand?" He looked at them like he wanted to ask "Understand WHAT?"

"Do you understand that we love you?" Dad's eyes glistened and tears rolled down his cheeks. Mom and Yossi were crying like babies.

When my two other brothers came back from their "mental treatment" and saw Yossi, Mom, and Dad crying, they thought that something terrible had happened. When they all got the picture, Yehuda went out and literally dropped to the hallway floor, sobbing to let out all his tension. Raffi sat down next to him, holding and hugging our oldest brother.

No words can ever really describe the feelings and intense emotions during these moments.

Raffi ran to the ICU to tell the staff about how alert my Dad was. One of the nurses started laughing and told Raffi that just before the transfer Dad *had talked* to her and asked: "Do you think that I will ever be able to make babies again?"

My Dad's sense of humor had returned to him as soon as he had opened his eyes.

It was just unbelievable. As she laughed her head off, the nurse told Raffi that she had answered my father:

"Maybe grandchildren, Meir."

The big day we had all waited for had arrived. Dad was alive in every way possible. We were overwhelmed, and the only way to express it was by looking at him, by holding him, and by crying.

He reacted the same way and we all exploded with happiness.

Chapter 19
A Letter to Dad

Back in Canada, across the seas and many miles away, I was wondering if Dad was missing me and my children. Was he asking himself where his daughter was? Did he remember his two lovely granddaughters in Canada?

I was hoping that he felt that he had been given the support he needed from our side of the Atlantic, but I was also worried that he was upset at us for being away from him when he needed us.

I felt then that it was the right time for me to take advantage of modern technology and use the communication tools available to us in the Internet age. I decided to send Yossi an e-mail that could be printed out and taken to my father. Communication systems had become so advanced that I couldn't remember the last time I had sent or received a hand-written letter or postcard. In the twenty-first century, when you send a fax or an e-mail out, it arrives almost instantaneously at its destination.

To my dear and most beloved Daddy,

If you only knew how much I miss you …

I wish I could be at your side, right now. My heart is torn apart.

Michal and Shiri have a difficult time accepting what has happened to you. They miss you very much, and are thinking of you all the time. When you will get stronger, and your breathing will be easier, we are going to tell you all that has happened and what we went through. Likewise, when you will be able to talk, we want to know what you have experienced.

I have so many things to say, and so many questions to ask you.

I am keeping a journal so I won't forget even the smallest detail. That way I will be able to tell you about everything that has gone on around you in the hospital. I can't wait to read it to you and Mom.

Daddy, I am far away across the ocean, but my heart and soul are with you every second. I have a hard time functioning at home and at work, but I learned from you to try and give my best, even through the most difficult times. I comfort myself by the fact that I know that Mom, Yehuda, Raffi, and Yossi are doing everything in their ability to take care of your needs and comfort. It is so inspiring to see their unity. It warms my heart.

I have no doubt Daddy that you are going through a very tough time, but your fight is absolutely worthy. Your will to live will win because you are strong and we are all beside you.

We need you.

I can't wait to talk with you on the phone and to see you.

You are surrounded by a very loving family that is just crazy about you, and I am SO proud of you. Do you want to know why I am so proud of you? I need lots of time to tell you, so get ready because I am already making all the preparations needed to come to Israel again. Very soon, I will be with you, to hold you, to hug you, and of course, to give you a headache ...

You need to recover fast, because I am dying to read my journal to you and Mom.

With all the love possible ...

A million hugs and kisses ...

Your only daughter,

Nechama

Up to this day, I am proud and happy to be the only girl in the family. When my baby brother Yossi was born, I was overjoyed to hear he was a boy so that my title of being the only girl was not taken from me.

Yossi printed the e-mail and brought it to the hospital the next day, but Dad was too sleepy and weak to be able to read it.

My letter would have to wait for a better day.

Chapter 20
Family Visits

Five weeks had passed from the day of the accident, and Yehuda was still going home only about once a week. He had not returned to work, had used up all his vacation days, and was on leave without pay. I was worried about him. He didn't see his family and hadn't resumed any of his regular daily activities. I spoke with him and suggested that he go back to work, at least on a part-time basis. Yehuda listened to me impatiently and said: "Okay, okay!" but, of course, continued on his way.

He needed to be in control of the situation every second of every day.

Mom also wanted to be on top of things *all* the time. She was at her husband's side every minute, and we tried to persuade her that this was going to do her more harm than good in the long run. Finally, after a lot of arguing, we were able to convince her that there was no need to stay all night at the hospital, especially since Yehuda promised to drive her back very early every morning.

He was very good at talking Mom and my brothers into getting back to their daily routines. Unfortunately, he wasn't so good at taking his own advice.

* * *

Now that Dad was in a regular unit, he could have family visits a few times a day. When Yossi came, he would often bring his lovely wife Keren, who was at that time in an advanced stage of pregnancy. As she came to visit, my dad used to greet her with a wide smile on his face while he gently touched her growing rounded belly. This was her first pregnancy, and on one of their visits Keren told him that they were going to have a girl they would name Danielle. We all felt that Yossi and Keren would be wonderful parents, but none of us knew their child would be a girl. My dad was actually first to get the news, and was very proud because Keren had honoured him before telling the rest of us.

Dad wasn't talking yet, but loved the family visits. He welcomed everyone with a smile, although that was all he could do as he was still extremely weak. This weakness also meant that he lost patience very quickly, so we asked our extended family to limit their stay to about fifteen minutes at a time. He had no energy, although he appreciated whoever came to see him.

There was one visitor that Dad loved and never got tired of. He was always so happy to see his grandson, Yaniv, Yehuda's son. Yaniv was a very gentle, quiet, and sensitive teenager. He used to come in, sit on Dad's bedside, come as close as possible to his grandpa, and hold his hand. Dad, very tenderly, would caress his "Yanivi's" head and kiss him.

During one of his visits, Yaniv ran out to the hallway as if a storm had hit the room. Nobody understood what was going on.

Yehuda went out and found him crying.

The two young men, father and son, stood there hugging tight and close as tears flowed on their faces. They cried out of the excitement they felt, witnessing their father and grandfather on the road to recovery.

Chapter 21
Challenging Nights

Dad's first night without Mom at his bedside was a terrible experience. We discovered that the night nurses were neither merciful nor sympathetic. When my mother arrived in the morning, she received a very cold welcome from Dad, who was angry and annoyed that he had been left alone. A private caregiver working for another person told Mom that the patients often had to wait long hours until they were attended to. She also reported that Dad hadn't slept all night and had been in excruciating pain. The nurses and the doctor on duty had ignored his calls, and when the caregiver had tried to get help for him, they only got upset, telling her to mind her own business.

The same morning, Dad's fever went up again and was now at 38.5°C (101.3°F). Besides this, his hearing was a disaster as he couldn't make out a single sound.

Mom went looking for a doctor. She spent hours trying to find someone who wasn't too busy to talk. When she finally got an answer, she was told that both the hearing loss and the fever were side effects of one of the antibiotics he was still on.

I could accept the doctor's clarification on Dad's hearing because we had been told from the beginning that while it would probably return gradually, there could be permanent loss. We were not worried so much about that, but were very concerned about the fever going up. I totally disagreed with the doctor's explanation, as it was clear that Dad had an infection from an unknown source. That was the reason he was on antibiotics to begin with! What the doctor had said seemed merely dismissive and had thus only deepened my anxiety.

I called the hospital and insisted on speaking with the same doctor who had talked with my mom. I told him my thoughts and concerns and insisted upon an ENT (ear, nose, and throat) specialist consultation, even though I knew that Dad's hearing problem wasn't as threatening a condition as the unknown infection. Dad had never been seen by a specialist because everybody assumed that the hearing loss was a result of his medication's side- effect. I suggested that the problem could have been caused by something as simple as wax buildup. I mentioned this because experience had taught me that doctors sometimes get "locked" on an issue without thinking about the small things that can cause the same effects.

In this situation, the doctor merely brushed me off and told me that that was not important now.

"Well, it is to us as we are screaming in my Dad's ear and he still doesn't hear a thing. His roommates' families are complaining about our noisy attempts to communicate, so it is important, very important, to us," I insisted.

An hour later an ENT doctor checked my Dad. I was happy about that, but not about my wish that it was just a little "wax in the ear" problem. The diagnosis justified all that the doctor had said: it was the side-effect of his medication. My hope was gone. It was possible now that Dad would remain deaf for the rest of his life.

In the meantime, Mom was begging the nurses to transfer Dad to a chair, even if only for a short while. It was important for him to sit up, particularly for his lungs, skin, and morale. He needed to see the world from a sitting position and thereby feel more human. After a three-hour wait, the request was followed, and Dad was transferred with a lift and the assistance of a nurse and two orderlies.

After this humiliating delay, my poor mom found herself begging the nurse again. She needed Dad put back to bed, as he had begun suffering unbearable pain in his legs as soon as he was put in a sitting position. He was crying in agony. My mom knew that if she was going to ask to have him put back to bed after all the hassle, it would be a declaration of war. She had to think very carefully and choose her words in a diplomatic way.

However, nothing would have changed the nurse's reaction at that moment. My mom was treated as a nudnik[6] who didn't know if she was coming or going. Mom knew that worse was to follow, but Dad was crying and she didn't care for her pride now.

"Mrs. Surik," the nurse said, "we can't work like this. You asked that we take him out of bed. That's what we did, and after all the effort needed, you want us to put him back? It doesn't work like this here. He will need to sit until we have time to transfer him. Don't ask again; we will be here when we can."

Mom was helpless and Dad was crying like a baby. The nurses had treated Mom as if she was the source of the problem and had totally ignored Dad. They had not even bothered to talk with him or to try to assess his condition.

This incident was one of the most important lessons of my entire professional career. There is no way that I will *ever* treat family members of people under my care as "difficult people." I have heard clinical staff (of all levels) describe a relative as being "difficult." Usually they are only "difficult" because they care; because they demand services for their loved ones; and because they advocate for those who can't speak for themselves. After all, there are lots of complicated, complex cases that require extra

---

[6] A nudnik is a Yiddish expression for a persistently annoying person.

attention. Unfortunately, some doctors and nurses occasionally use their control and influence in a way that does not serve the best interests of the patient. While most health- care professionals are dedicated, caring people who give everything they can to their work, one act of selfish or ignorant behavior can undermine the trust of the patients and their families in the entire system.

The general public is aware of the shortage of clinical staff but can generally bear the frustration up to a certain point. Many conflicts that have been blamed on understaffing could be avoided by using proper communication skills. Health care is not just the most important aspect of public service — it is about our lives. I expect health care professionals to be compassionate, to listen and not just hear, and to serve the public by using their authority in a positive way. There is no need for a doctor's prescription to lend an ear or to share a smile, and there are definitely no side effects!

* * *

My mom wasn't lucky on that day; she suffered with Dad and was ripped to pieces inside. After a while she asked again: "Please, can you find a few moments to transfer my husband to bed? Look, he is crying; he can't take the pain."

"Mrs. Surik," said the nurse, "it's not a playground here, and we have many duties. It was you who insisted on transferring your husband to the chair, and although we were very busy, we answered your request. Now you will have to wait."

My mom had to wait? It wasn't my mother who had to wait, it was my father! He had no say in the situation and yet was being punished for my mom's "sin." All she could do was swallow her pride and bite her tongue. There was nothing more to be said.

When I heard the story, I was out of my mind in anger. The nurse could have changed the situation completely. She could have given the exact same message without deliberately hurting my mother simply by changing her tone of voice and by saying something like:

"Mrs. Surik, I understand, and it is a problem. We are very busy, so let me check to see if I can give Meir something for pain. In the meantime, sit next to him and talk with him. I promise you that as soon as I can, I will be back to get your husband to bed."

It's not what you say, but how you say it.

For two full hours my parents were sitting side by side and crying, Dad for the pain and Mom for Dad. When my father was finally transferred to bed, they were both exhausted and worn out. They were dead from the pain, but were even more battered emotionally. They had been completely drained from the humiliation they had to go through.

Chapter 22
The Israeli Medicare System

Despite the isolated problems my family experienced with certain individuals in the hospital, the Israeli health care system has some excellent features, an inclusive philosophy, and many dedicated and worthy practitioners. Over the last decade, Israeli scientific breakthroughs (especially in the high-tech field) have given the national health organization huge advantages. Many other countries have similar resources but have not applied them so imaginatively. In my opinion, the Israeli system represents a high standard in its approach to universal health care and thus can be used as a model around the globe.

Every Israeli citizen has the right to full, free health care and is issued a "Medicare" card, much like the Canadian model. While the Israeli card entitles its bearers to similar services available to Canadian residents, there are major differences in the way the two cards function.

The Israeli card is not just used as identification or as a billing tool for medical appointments and services. It gives every holder the right to fully control his or her quality of care. Each individual can access their medical history and updated information by logging in to the Internet or at easily-accessible public terminals. Test results are available to view within forty-eight hours without waiting for a physician's call or for another appointment and it is still the doctor's responsibility to notify the patient if there is something out of the ordinary that needs attention. Additionally, if one has to schedule an appointment to see a doctor or have a diagnostic test, it can be done on-line. There is no need to spend precious time listening to annoying voice mail messages. With the computerized system, the patient just logs in and sets up a meeting. Furthermore, when booking a test that requires preparation, there will be an automatic notification of all the information needed *specific to the test and to the individual's condition.*

For example, if you are going to undergo a blood test and need to abstain from foods and liquids, the computerized system will tell you how long you need to fast. If you suffer from hypertension, you will be instructed to take your blood pressure pills through your fast. The same thing applies for many other conditions as well (diabetes, allergies, etc.). If you still have questions, you can call a toll-free, twenty-four-hour hotline, and an authorized person will address your concerns.

Individuals that have no access to a computer are not left out in the cold; they also have a very easy way to obtain their health information. There is a machine, like a bank machine here, in most pharmacies and health clinics. At these terminals, you merely slide your Medicare card through the convenient port, enter your PIN, and all the information you need about your own health will be printed out for you. You can schedule your appointments the same way. Not only does this system provide people with total control, it also allows for better care, as doctors are more available to see their patients. GPs can often see you on the same day because they are not busy on the phone, and the average wait time for a specialist is less than two weeks. This also significantly reduces pressure on the ER, as people know that they can readily see their family physician. On the other hand, if someone chooses to go to the ER, they are automatically charged $20 per visit and get reimbursed only if the doctor can provide a certificate stating that the visit was indeed an emergency.

One of the most important innovations of the Israeli health care system is its recognition of alternative medicine. While many doctors still use conventional treatments, others have obtained licenses in alternative medicine and operate successful and thriving practices. Some have gone on to study both fields and work by combining the two disciplines, using techniques from each as appropriate to the individual needs of the patient.

The choices offered to the Israeli public in their health care system are positive, clinically and mentally. Many people in health systems that do not acknowledge alternative cures hide their use of holistic remedies from their family doctor. This problem can lead to situations in which regular medication can operate in contradiction to the "natural" products. The Israeli approach prevents this because of the integration of the alternative and conventional disciplines. As well, the integration itself mitigates conflict within the profession as well as between health care practitioners and their clients.

Finally, the choice between alternative or mainstream medicine is not limited to picking a doctor or between different types of medication. There are very popular alternative hospitals in Israel that are totally covered by public health insurance.

This is a win-win situation for everybody. The patients have much more control and choice, and the doctors have fewer anxious and frustrated clients. The result is a happier and healthier population. On the other hand, do not get the impression that there are no problems within the system. To get certain special medications that are not covered financially requires extreme patience. Israelis, not generally known for their patience, have another quality that assists them in these special circumstances. Their "Chutzpa" is famous for a reason ... it is how they bulldoze through the bureaucracy!

In September 2008 my mom had to undergo surgery, so I went to Israel to be at her bedside with my family. As she was transferred to the operating room, we were given a piece of paper with a code number on it. We were instructed that this number, along with others, would be displayed on a big electronic flat screen TV in the waiting room. Beside each code there was a line of text which read: "waiting for surgery" or "in the recovery room" etc. The information was clear and easy to follow and we didn't need to wait anxiously without knowing what was going on. The code number given to us was designed to maintain privacy; a different one was assigned to every patient, so that relatives could confidentially follow their loved ones' progress. This very simple computerized system was a huge help for the OR personnel, because it allowed them to spend time with the patients instead of attending stressed family members. People no longer needed to line up at the OR door, because they now had the updated information in real time.

During the same visit to Israel, I went to have a talk with one of my dad's doctors. My mom gave me my dad's Medicare card (along with the PIN number) and told me to simply slide it in the machine located at the clinic entrance. My sixty-nine year old mom, who doesn't know how to turn on a computer, explained in seconds how to operate this advanced system: "Just slide the card across, enter the PIN, and you will know everything." She was right! I instantly received a "print out" that stated the particulars of my father's appointment: his name, the name of his doctor, the floor and room number I should go to, and even how long the line-up was. When I got to the office, the doctor's door was open. As he didn't know me and expected to see my dad, he was surprised and asked if I had an appointment. After I explained to him that I was here on behalf of Meir Surik he responded:

"Oh, that's great. I had no more appointments, but I was waiting here because I saw that the card had been activated and I knew that you had come into the building."

I couldn't believe it. The system really worked!

Chapter 23
Pressure Sores

Five weeks after Dad was hospitalized, Yossi told me that our father had a huge buttocks (coccyx) pressure sore. It was no surprise but certainly a significant worry.

Pressure sores form as a result of prolonged pressure or constant rubbing of one particular spot on the body. The key to dealing with this problem is *prevention*.

Every institution has protocols to prevent pressure sores from occurring, and these are basic and universal for nursing practice. If these rules are respected, the problem will be radically reduced. Some of these practices include: changing the patients' position every two hours, keeping sensitive areas clean and dry, and maintaining a well-balanced diet and good hydration. Additionally, there are a variety of mattresses designed to address this issue that can be recommended by physiotherapists and occupational therapists.

If protocols are not followed, or if preventive measures fail, pressure sores will result. These can develop very quickly, but unfortunately take a much longer period of time to heal. While they cause enormous discomfort, suffering, and pain, the most significant risk they pose is through the formation of local or systemic infections. In these cases, treatments by different dressing applications and techniques are used. In more serious circumstances, local or systemic medications, including antibiotics, are sometimes prescribed, and in the worst situations surgical intervention may be necessary.

I was actually surprised that Dad had only one pressure sore because the nature of his injury did not allow the frequent position changes which would otherwise prevent formation of these dangerous wounds.

Sure enough, just two days after we found out about the first sore, we discovered that Dad had another big, ugly lesion at the back of his head, due to his prolonged bedridden state. Now we had another thing to worry about, and everybody in my family had good reason to be anxious.

Chapter 24
An Unpredictable September

Time had passed by filled with ups and downs; the changes were often dramatic from one day to the next. It looked as if Dad had lost his hearing completely, but then he started to demonstrate indications of recovery. The first signal was his whispered complaints. It was actually nice to hear him kvetching, but it was no surprise, as his fever was still 38.5°C (101.3°F), and he didn't feel good at all. The doctor maintained his confidence and stuck to his opinion that the fever was a side effect of the antibiotics.

One morning, Dad started perspiring abnormally. This was not good news.

A sudden drop of his blood pressure (80/40) was the cause. The doctors asked all visitors to leave the room, and as they were busy with their diagnosis, Yossi called to put me in the picture. He thought that due to the deterioration in Dad's condition, I should be ready in case he needed to return to the ICU. My brother was right. In less than an hour, Dad was back in the ICU, anaesthetized and on a respirator. He was in critical condition, and his life was in danger again.

The mood was intense and brutal, and we were all devastated. Everyone walked around with fallen faces and anguished hearts. It was tough to accept the situation when we already had seen some signs of recovery. We had even begun to think about rehab, and then without warning, like a lightning strike out of a clear sky, everything collapsed with a huge crash.

Now, Dad's recovery seemed further away than ever.

My father had acute life-threatening pneumonia, and the idea that the fever was a result of an antibiotic side-effect was not only purely speculative, it was extremely dangerous, because the real problem was not treated. This infection could have put any healthy person's life in jeopardy, so there was no question that Dad's life was again on the line. I can't describe how I felt. I was so angry at the doctor, and felt cheated and betrayed by his ignorance. All the way through, his diagnosis hadn't made sense to me, but he had demonstrated so much confidence that I felt I had no choice but to go along. Despite knowing in my heart that it was not possible, I kind of 'wanted to believe' what he had been insisting over and over. Now, I also felt guilty for accepting his explanations. Above all, I was worried to death, and like the rest of my family, feared for my father's life.

The ICU staff, who knew us all and who had already witnessed the many hardships we had gone though, was supportive, warm, and compassionate throughout this new emergency.

Contrary to the first time Dad was in the ICU (when the general strategy was to withhold positive information in order to avoid crushing disappointments), the team was very encouraging; they assured us that they would be able to overcome the crisis and that "everything would be okay." As we all fully and completely trusted the ICU personnel, we felt we could depend on that statement. It was the only source of hope that we could cling to.

All the necessary tests were taken and were sent to the lab to figure out what kind of parasite had attacked Dad. The next step was to find the bacteria's sensitivity so that we could destroy it before it killed him. While they were busy identifying the bacteria in the lab, I was busy booking a seat on an El Al flight. I wanted to leave as soon as possible and started arranging time off work. I was able to get a ticket for October 30, 2000.

I had been impatiently looking forward to this visit and had endured many long, sleepless nights in the process. Now I was going to see my family again, and with great anticipation, hoped to see my father responsive and awake.

Chapter 25
Politics

A few days passed and Dad began to recover thanks to the effective antibiotic treatment. Then the process of slow and gradual withdrawal from his respiratory machine and the anesthesia began all over again. To our surprise, and unlike the previous time, Dad immediately showed signs of alertness after the dosage of his medication was decreased. He began to pronounce words and even voiced short sentences.

During Dad's fourth day in the intensive care unit, Mom sat next to him and held his hand as hard as she possibly could.

Suddenly, Dad whispered:

"You are a good woman."

Mom was excited by the sound of his voice and replied that he was the best husband in the world and that she loved him. He looked at her, lowered his gaze past his legs, and told her:

"I want to die."

These words broke Mom's spirit. She called me and exploded in a heart-wrenching cry as she repeated what he had said. While it was also difficult for me to hear about Dad's suffering, I tried to encourage her:

"It is natural that he feels this way," I said.

"At least he recognizes you, talks to you, and shares his pain with you. Together we shall help him to overcome his suffering, and you more than anyone. He needs you, Mom, more than anybody else in the world. It is thanks to you that he is alive. He is here because of your hands holding him. He is still with us because of your presence, devotion, and love. He did not imply that you are a good woman for no reason. He is aware of everything that you are doing."

These words encouraged and empowered Mom and gave her the strength to return to his side.

* * *

A day later, on September 15, Dad began to smile and say logical sentences, even though there was no improvement in his hearing.

The same day he asked:

"How is Nechama?"

Due to Dad's deafness, Raffi had to raise his voice to explain that I was in Canada yet that I had spent many hours with him over the past month. Dad replied with a facial expression, which implied, "I know." No one understood the meaning of his reaction and before we could begin to process it, he asked:

"Who is the prime-minister?"

Yossi provided Dad with a short political briefing. He told him that Ehud Barak was the prime-minister and that Arie Dery had been incarcerated. A big smile came to Dad's face, revealing his satisfaction. Yossi did not conceal the more unpleasant news from our father: within the same week, a difficult situation had arisen in the occupied territories. Rocks were being thrown at Israeli soldiers, and our men had responded with fire. The situation was extremely serious, as eighty Arabs from the territories had been killed by the IDF.[7] Besides this, within the Lebanese border, three of our soldiers were killed; an event which agitated the whole country. Barak gave a speech to the United Nations, declaring a forty-eight-hour ultimatum to stop the uprising. The prime-minister proclaimed that if the measures didn't work, Israeli military activities would be intensified. The whole world fearfully followed what was going on, and Bill Clinton, the president of United States, prepared for a visit to Israel.

---

[7] Israeli Defense Forces

Everybody prayed that a war would not erupt, and I was crossing my fingers hoping for a cease-fire. Of course, I wanted this for Israel's benefit but also for the most selfish of reasons:

I was hoping that the airport would be open for landings and that I would be able to see Dad on October 30 as planned.

Chapter 26
Rejoicing

Rosh Hashanah (the Jewish New Year) had passed without much notice, as we did not feel the holiday spirit. Nevertheless, I sent Mom and Dad my blessings and love for a happy and sweet new year. This year's wishes carried particular significance.

Soon after, Yom Kippur's[8] eve arrived, and because of his medical condition, my father was fasting. This was slightly humorous, as he had never paid attention to the holidays or the Jewish religious laws. While not allowed to eat, he was fed with the aid of a nasogastric feeding tube (a tube which passes through the nostrils and descends into the stomach). If the doctors only knew Dad's thoughts regarding Yom Kippur, they would have given him steak through the tube! We laughed at the fact that Dad was urged to break "his" tradition and was unable to have a meal on Yom Kippur.

The next day, the feeding tube was removed. Raffi and Ayelet arrived that night along with a meal to "break the fast." They cautiously fed Dad macaroni. He ate the meal with a big appetite, just like those who had

---

[8] *Yom Kippur*, the *Day of Atonement*, is the most solemn and important of the Jewish holidays. Jews have traditionally observed this holiday with a twenty-four-hour period of fasting and intensive prayer.

performed their religious duties by abstaining from food on the "Day of Atonement."

* * *

During the next two days, Dad's body temperature rose and was bouncing between 38° and 39°C (100.4° to 102.2°F). The excessively high fever undoubtedly signified a problem. The staff sat him up on a chair for several hours, but despite his high temperature, he seemed happy and did not complain about any discomfort or pain. Mom felt better seeing Dad at peace.

I took advantage of the "good day" and phoned Israel, asking my mother to devote some time to herself. Since Dad had returned to the intensive care unit, Mom had not slept at home. I felt that it was time for her to spend a few nights in her own bed and to return to the hospital during the later hours of the day. Things could not proceed as before. I tried to convince her by telling her that she must take care of herself in order to take care of Dad. To my surprise, she agreed. To me, this was proof that she was exhausted and beginning to lose her physical strength.

The following night, Mom slept at home. The next day she called me and reported that my father had greeted her with an angry expression, asking her if she was too bored and fed up to sit by his side. He also cynically questioned whether it was too much for her to pay for a private nurse to sit with him while Mom was away. This was a clear sign that Dad was fully conscious. He knew exactly which buttons to push in order to make his wife feel guilty. Before, when Mom had stayed in the hospital, Dad did not want to let her go home even though hospital policy forbade her inside his room. As a result, she lost her strength without actually being able to spend the night at his side.

While the way my father had acted was extremely selfish, it was quite typical for people in his condition. He did not intend to hurt her feelings or aggravate the situation. It was simply a reaction to his great pain and distress and arose from the fear of his own mortality.

Mom, who had finally enjoyed a night's sleep in her own bed, decided that she could no longer give in to her husband's pressure tactics. She looked into private nursing services and made arrangements for someone to be with him at night after he was transferred to the regular unit. I was proud of her wise decision. Setting limits is a difficult task, especially for my mom, who all her life did everything to please Dad.

Chapter 27
Hallucinations

Time passed. I continued to get constant updates, as I had in the first days of the accident. I heard what each doctor had said; how high the blood pressure was; how much urine was in the catheter bag; whether he had a fever; the level of oxygen in the blood; the pain control; and, of course, Dad's general mood. Fortunately, each day brought a significant improvement, and Dad was transferred from the ICU back to the "refugee camp." The place was still crowded, bustling and uncomfortable. According to Raffi, compared to the ICU, Dad's stay in this department was like "sleeping on the ground without a sheet."

Dad had started breathing independently and now only needed the assistance of the respirator a few times a day. At this point, my family started back to their regular routines and gradually returned both to work and to spending time with their wives and children.

That same year, the Olympic Games took place in Australia. Yossi kept telling me that he hoped that the Canadian athletes would not win any competition or game. I did not understand why he said those things and asked him why he was so mad at Canada. His answer was that of an angry child. He explained to me that if Canada had never existed, I would be with my family in Israel rather than so far away. They say the young always speak the truth; Yossi sounded just like a little child who was honestly expressing his feelings. This reaction, from someone who was soon to become a father, was very touching to me.

* * *

My flight ticket was dated for October 30, 2000, and lay next to my passport. It was over a month since the accident and Dad was fully conscious, although his hearing had not yet improved. Despite being completely deaf, he had learned how to express himself very efficiently. His sense of humor was back, along with his many cynical expressions not particularly pleasant to functional ears. Just to mention one example: Once, when Yehuda went out for a smoke, as he did every short while, Dad asked him sarcastically:

"Tell me Yehuda, did you come to visit me or Marlboro?"

Everyone exploded with laughter, although I'm not sure if Yehuda enjoyed the joke.

We had been waiting with great anticipation for Dad to return to full consciousness, but there was a downside to his recovery. Around the same time as he awoke to what was going on around him, he began to suffer side effects from the narcotics used during his long period of anesthetization. The worst of these were the hallucinations. We thought we knew what to expect because we were warned by the doctors and had heard from others who had experienced them. However, nothing could have prepared us for what Dad went through ... and for what we went through along with him.

There are many types of hallucination: visual, auditory, and olfactory to name but a few. They are all complicated to deal with, since they seem completely real to the person experiencing them.

My dad had "fantasy" hallucinations in which he was actually totally awake but was imagining an entirely different situation than what was apparent to those around him. He described everything in his imaginary world, lived the experience, and showed all the emotions of being part of it. When we would attempt to explain what "reality" was, we met with failure, because for him reality was only what he had experienced.

Dad's hallucinations were one of the most difficult things Mom had to face. He was often mad at her, accusing her of making "deals;" bribing the doctors to prevent her from visiting so that she could stay at home instead of being next to him. He even accused her of having affairs with *all* the doctors.

Mom would burst into tears on hearing these claims and had a lot of difficulty facing this problem. She couldn't function normally, and while the rest of us saw her lose control, we couldn't do anything about it. After a particularly strange outburst from Dad, she would be afraid to come in the next day because she didn't know what would be going on in his head.

Yossi told me that Dad hallucinated that I was hiding out around the hospital, sleeping somewhere far away from him. When he had been asked what had made him think that, he said that I had been late for the "boat" back to Canada, and that instead of sitting next to him until the next "boat" arrived, I had wanted to keep my distance.

It was a horrific, frightening experience. We just hoped that the doctors were right and that his mental state would soon return to normal. We knew that Mom couldn't bear it for too much longer, and that without some relief, the rest of us would end up in the "mental ward" as well.

Often the hallucinations would last for many hours. When they were over, Dad would not remember a thing.

Aside from his endless "fantasies," Dad's deafness and speech difficulties (due to the tracheotomy) caused Yehuda and Raffi to feel helpless. They could barely communicate with him at all, and this drove them nuts. Only Mom and Yossi could understand what he was saying, and they were the only ones able to explain things to him when he was in a reasonable state of mind.

Raffi found Dad's "visions" especially hard to take and tried to stay away from the crazy situation as much as possible. He occupied himself by running through the hallways of government, taking care of the many complex, bureaucratic issues related to the accident. We were all very grateful that he took that burden off our shoulders.

As we each dealt with this crisis in our own way, we all hoped that Dad's "hallucinatory" state would one day become a source of laughter, and even a way to tease him. At that point, it wasn't funny at all.

Chapter 28
Back to Israel

When Dad heard that I had a plane ticket to Israel at hand, he started marking Xs on the calendar Yossi had prepared especially for this purpose. He had something to look forward to, as did the rest of my family, who needed my help. Mom was tired from her long, sleepless nights, and the day-to-day tension was leaving everyone totally exhausted.

On the other hand, Dad did not show any concern or agony over his amputated leg. He knew that he would eventually be fitted with a prosthesis, so his approach was very positive. He just wanted to be pain free.

My father's acceptance of his new reality was so complete and relaxed that once, when Yaniv came for a visit, Dad told him: "Yanivi, as soon as I get out of the hospital with a new leg, I will go to a soccer game with you."

I impatiently waited for the date Dad had clearly marked in his "countdown calendar"- the date of my arrival in Israel. Twenty-four hours prior to the flight, I was unable to eat or sleep at all. The anticipation and excitement were enormous. I was going to see my family again!

On October 31, I was walking on the pathway leading to the Ichilov Hospital once more.

I got there in the evening, directly from the airport. I was led to the "refugee camp," where Dad waited for me in his bed, filled with anticipation, He had a large bandage wrapped around his head covering the enormous bedsore he had at the time. The moment I saw my father alive and smiling was tremendously emotional. Tears immediately filled our eyes. I had been waiting for this for so long! Mom seemed very tired, and she had lost a lot of weight. The three months she spent at the hospital were showing on her beautiful face. It was so wonderful to hug Mom and tell her:

"Go home to sleep. From now on, and for as long as I'm here, you will be sleeping at home."

It was tough for Dad to let Mom go, although he gave his approval to pass the "shift" to me. It was obvious that he was very happy to see me and that he trusted me completely.

Dad still suffered from a lot of pain. The night prior to my arrival he had received extra doses of pain killers, but these had given him only a little relief over a very short period of time. I gazed at him for long hours with concern, yet filled with an immense pride. I asked myself how a person could go through so much—such horrible pain, tubes penetrating every possible part of their body, and furthermore having to bear this while almost completely immobile. Where did Dad draw all his strength?

I was at my father's bedside for practically an entire month, and only left the hospital occasionally, in order to shower and to sleep on a real bed for a few hours.

The nights were tough. Dad began trying to pull out every accessible tube connected to his body. He knew what he was going to do and would wait until I looked away for an instant. When I scratched my nose, it was time to carry out the mission! I was forced to stay up and be ready to jump when Dad was up to this kind of mischief. I begged him not to do this and was very mad when he succeeded. I tried to explain to him that the pain would be much worse when the doctors were forced to prick his veins again.

One night, after I got especially upset, Dad said to me: "I know you are disappointed and angry at me. In fact, so much so, that I don't feel the same warmth from you as when you got here."

I burst into tears. I tried to explain to him how proud I was and yet how worried I was for his health at the same time. How could I explain to him that in my eyes he was simply a hero? Only heroes can hang on and even keep a sense of humor in this situation.

Like the hero he was, Dad said many funny things in between his moments of pain. Once, when I went to the bathroom in the middle of the night, he asked a doctor who happened to be passing through:

"Did you see my daughter?"

"Yes" the doctor answered. "I saw her walking toward the bathroom."

"For so long?" Dad asked.

"Meir, are you timing how long she's gone to the bathroom?"

"Sure," Dad answered with a straight face and without hesitation.

When I came back from the bathroom, the doctor was standing at the room entrance and said: "You better have a pretty good explanation as to why it took three whole minutes to return." I sat next to Dad and waited for him to say something. He held my hands warmly, as if he wanted to ask me not to leave him alone. That's how we sat together the entire night.

Every morning, between 7:00 and 10:00 a.m., all visitors were asked to exit the rooms so the doctors could do their rounds, examining and treating their patients. During that time, I used to stretch out on a bench in the hospital's backyard, as if I was homeless, and take a short nap outside. I would completely ignore everything around me. When I'd return to the room, I would find my mom already there, waiting to be let in.

* * *

Another month had passed, and Dad was feeling better and better. The tube feeding and the catheter were both removed, and he finally no longer needed the breathing machine. The tracheostomy opening was being reduced each day, and his speech was much clearer and easier to understand as a result. There was even an improvement in hearing.

On the other hand, my father was getting more picky. For one, he would only agree to eat Mom's food. Each day, she would bring whole baskets filled with the delicious dishes she had cooked the previous day, excluding morning porridge. Dad would not touch "hospital food." Mom had spoiled him with her scrumptious food for many years, but now she cooked more than ever because she wanted her "Tzuptzik" to get stronger and to put on weight. The Halvah hidden at the bottom of the basket was the "secret" ingredient in ensuring her husband's return to "health!" Dad began complaining about many other things too, which we all took as a good sign. A sign he was getting better.

* * *

The doctors started talking about rehabilitation. Yehuda drove with Mom, Raffi, and Yossi to check out various hospitals around the country. I really hoped Dad would move to one while I was still in Israel so that I'd be able to see him start the rehab process.

At last, my departure date arrived. On exactly the same day, the doctors announced that Dad would be moving to a rehab hospital. What a celebration! Knowing Dad was going to get out of the hospital after four torturous months was a gift to me. He glowed with happiness, just like the rest of us. I was sitting next to him as usual when he suddenly asked a surprising question:

"Nechamale," he called me as always, "I don't understand how it could be that when I was in intensive care, you were always next to me each time I opened my eyes. Day and night. Any hour. How was that possible? I know it was not one of my hallucinations."

I was stunned.

"Dad, you want to tell me that when I was next to you in the ICU, you knew that I was there?"

Dad knew and remembered many things that totally amazed me. He would describe to me how I bathed him, how I massaged his legs and arms, and how I had talked to him. I was so concerned that my father hadn't been aware of my presence, and yet he remembered things I had said to him while there was no one else in the room. There was no way anyone was able to tell him what I had said, so it was obvious that he had been conscious at the time.

Now, while I had always believed it was wrong to talk about an unconscious patient as if they weren't there (as many professionals and family members unfortunately tend to do), my opinion on the matter only got stronger. My father had "opened my eyes" to his high level of awareness, even while he was under the most powerful drugs.

I said goodbye to everyone with mixed feelings. I had wanted to stay with Mom and Dad during the rehab, which I knew would be very difficult. This time, however, I was leaving with a big smile on my face. Dad was in a totally different state than he was in the last time I had returned to Canada. I knew that he would be transferred within days and that he did not think I was abandoning him. Most of all, I knew that he realized that I was proud of him to the skies.

Chapter 29
Rehab

Several days after my return to Montreal, Dad and the entire family said goodbye to the staff in the Ichilov hospital. It was an emotional farewell, for they were the ones who had been taking such dedicated care of him for so many long months and who were really responsible for saving his life. Thanks to them, this long-awaited and joyful day was finally here. Dad was transferred to the Beith Rivka rehab hospital in Petach Tikva. An ambulance was required because of his physical condition, but there were no sirens in the background this time, and it was a very calm and comfortable drive.

However this was not the end of my dad's ordeal: a new battle was about to begin.

Although his life was no longer in immediate danger, there were still many drastic ups and downs during his stay in Beith Rivka. He often had to travel back and forth to the Ichilov hospital to treat various fever-causing infections. His struggle continued moment by moment, day by day.

As Dad began receiving physiotherapy treatment, the initial focus was on his upper extremities, as his leg muscles were too weak after so many long months in bed. This meant that in order to function independently on a basic level, his arms first needed to gain strength. Despite his frailty, he learned how to use the wheelchair, to self-transfer from the wheelchair to bed and back, and to use the bathroom on his own. Unfortunately, since he still suffered from breathing complications, physical activity was much more difficult, and besides slowing his recovery, this also necessitated many more medical procedures.

* * *

Aside from these complaints, Dad always kept his sense of humor, even through the worst treatments. He worked very hard and gradually started to get stronger. Mom would not miss a single day, coming to Beith Rivka each morning and only leaving at night. My brothers were back at work, so she had to use public transportation. Even traveling by bus, she would carry full baskets of the delicious dishes she made for her spoiled "Tzuptzik," as he would go on "a hunger strike" otherwise. Each day on her way home, Mom would go grocery shopping and then cook fresh food (God forbid Dad would eat the same dish twice in a row!). After a long day of traveling and spending time at the hospital, we all would wonder where she got her strength.

There is a Hebrew expression: "Who can find a wonder woman?" Well, my father certainly did!

* * *

Dad began putting on weight from eating the food Mom made for him, which pleased her to no end. Months passed, and he was told that he would soon receive a customized prosthetic leg. He was looking forward to the day he would be able to stand on both feet and dance with his wife again. He had been a wonderful step dancer, with movements as light as a professional's.

One day, the physiotherapist notified Dad that his "leg" had arrived from the factory. The prosthesis was ready and there was enormous excitement. The entire staff grouped all around my father in order to witness his first step. After it was strapped on, he lifted himself with the help of the physiotherapist and his walker. Dad was standing on both legs for the first time since the accident! Everyone without exception was moved to tears as they finally saw Dad on his feet. The orderlies, the nurses, the doctors, and all who were watching enthusiastically cheered for him. Mom was eternally happy. We had been waiting for this day for so long … and now Dad was standing with his head high. He knew that if he wanted to return home, he had to function independently. With enormous effort he had taken the "first step" on that journey.

Slowly, step by step, he learned to walk with his prosthetic leg. This process was accompanied by a lot of pain, varying moods, extreme efforts, and much encouragement from his caregivers. While we all cheered him on as much as possible, the real effort was up to him. Dad missed the home he shared with Mom very much and worked hard to get there. After learning to use the wheelchair, he would roll down to the elevator every day to greet Mom. Sometimes he would even go downstairs to the backyard and wait for her there. He would always look at his watch and check if she was late; if she was, he refused to go to his physiotherapy session without her. Even though she would get mad at him for not going, she was also happy that he wanted her constant presence.

* * *

Beith Rivka is a very warm place thanks to its wonderful and dedicated personnel. Their long, intensive, everyday work with Dad was indeed fruitful, and after many hours and days of therapy, the decision was reached that he was ready to go back home.

A team of professionals was sent to my parents' apartment in order to assess whether it fit my father's new needs. They recommended a few vital changes which had to be made immediately: the removal of some walls to allow passage for the wheelchair and alterations in the layout of the bathroom. My brothers took immediate action, and all the advised modifications were made.

My parents were about to embark on the next chapter in their lives!

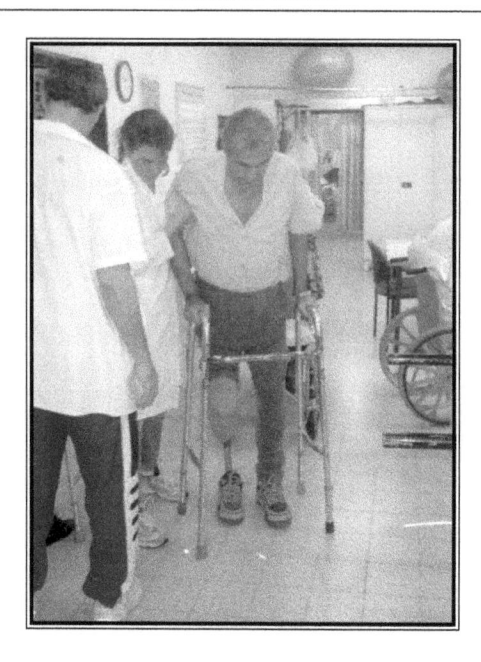

The first step with the prosthesis.

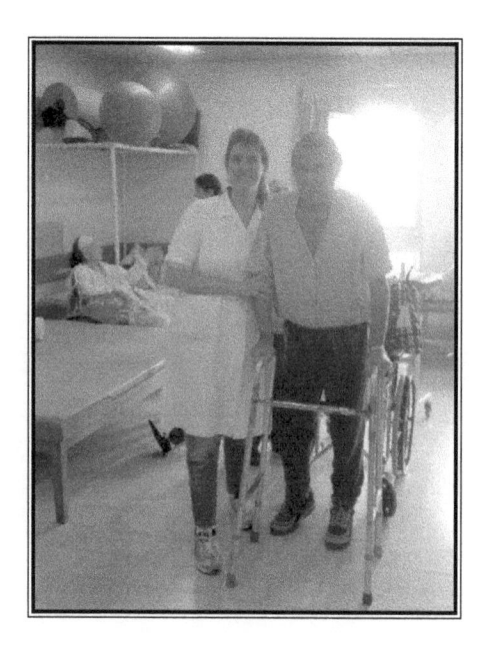

Dad learning to walk again with the help of his devoted physiotherapist.

Chapter 30
The Return Home

In July, 2001, nearly a year after the accident, my dad finally returned home. We were all still worried, as there was no elevator in the building my parents were living in. In order to reach their apartment, Dad would have to climb up twenty-two steps—a difficult task for a person suffering from a chronic lung disease (COPD), and doubly difficult for my father. Although the action of climbing the stairs was practiced each day in Beith Rivka, we were not sure how Dad would deal with whatever other unforeseen obstacles he might have to face.

My parents arrived home on a Thursday afternoon, and the entire family was frantically following each step Dad made as he climbed the stairs leading to the entrance of the apartment. He went up slowly, holding the side railing, and took only one break in the middle of the journey to inhale some oxygen into his lungs. As a big, winning smile was smeared all over his face, he walked forward. What an emotional moment! Little less than a year earlier, Dad had left for work. No one had ever imagined it would take so long for his return.

Minutes later my phone rang in Montreal. I was no longer afraid to answer it; I was waiting for Dad to call, and I picked up the receiver immediately. "Nechamale, I'm back!" he said, and we both cried.

Even today it is hard to describe the relief I felt, knowing Dad was calling from home and that Mom no longer had to go back and forth to the hospital.

As my parents started adjusting to their new reality, it became obvious they would have to move to a different place. Their four-bedroom suite was large and comfortable, but the stairs were a serious problem. Climbing these in days when Dad did not feel at his best was a major challenge, which also left my mom uneasy. For this reason, he often stayed at home.

Their condo was put up for sale, and I promised to come and help them look for a new one. In September 2001, I arrived to help, and it was a delight for me to spend this time with them. Although they had already sold their old place, they managed to hold onto it until after I arrived, and a later moving date was agreed upon in order for us to be able to look without further pressure. I woke up early each day to go "home-hunting" and would only return in the evening. There was not a single real estate agent in town who did not know me, and there was not a sole vacancy in Rehovot I did not see.

It was agreed that we would be looking for a two-bedroom apartment to make the maintenance of the house easier on my mom. I also knew that if I was to find an apartment above ground level, an elevator would be necessary. There were a few other non-negotiable considerations I had to keep in mind as well: easy wheelchair access and an open-space style floor arrangement.

This mission was more complicated than I had initially thought. As it turned out, many elevators were just too narrow for a wheelchair. For this reason, the first thing I did going house-hunting, was to measure the entrance size of the elevator.

I went looking about town for many days, but only took my parents to see the most likely properties. Just two days prior to my return to Canada, I found an apartment that I immediately fell in love with. I brought my parents to see it and they felt the same. It was a recently constructed two-bedroom unit in a high-rise, located in a new area in Rehovot. Although it was on the second floor, the building included a suitable elevator. In fact, all accesses to the building were wheelchair-friendly. There was an open-space kitchen in the apartment, and the sink and the countertop were not too high. This was very important, as it enabled Dad to reach the tap while sitting in the wheelchair. Finally, there was a central air-conditioning system and a nice balcony.

Mom and Dad arranged to sign the contract on the day I left. My brothers were very pleased that I took responsibility for all the apartment-related issues. Although I asked them to go see the chosen home before signing the contract (to check all final details I might have missed), they said they trusted my instincts completely and that the most important thing was that our parents were pleased with the choice.

I went back home with a good feeling. While my brothers only saw the flat on moving day, they were very happy with it. They moved Mom and Dad a few months later, and everything went smoothly.

* * *

My parents had begun a new chapter in their lives. They had a new home, a new shopping area, new neighbors, and a new health clinic: everything was new. They enjoyed it all, even though their apartment was significantly smaller than their old one.

Dad continued his physiotherapy sessions at home with the aid of a professional. He learned how to use crutches and started walking with them in the house as well as outside. We were all so proud when he took his first trip downtown alone on the bus.

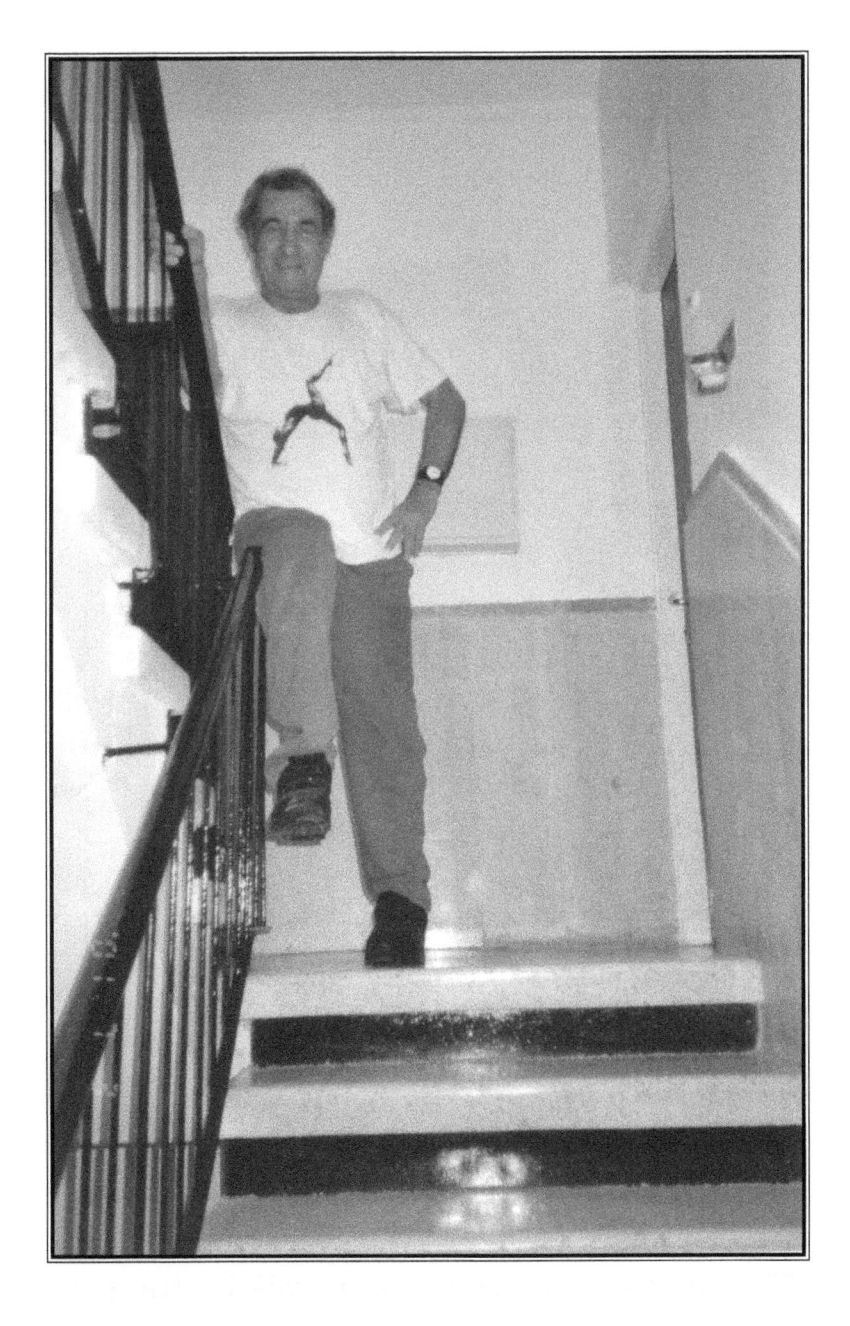

The victory picture: Dad in the stairway of the old house on the first day home.

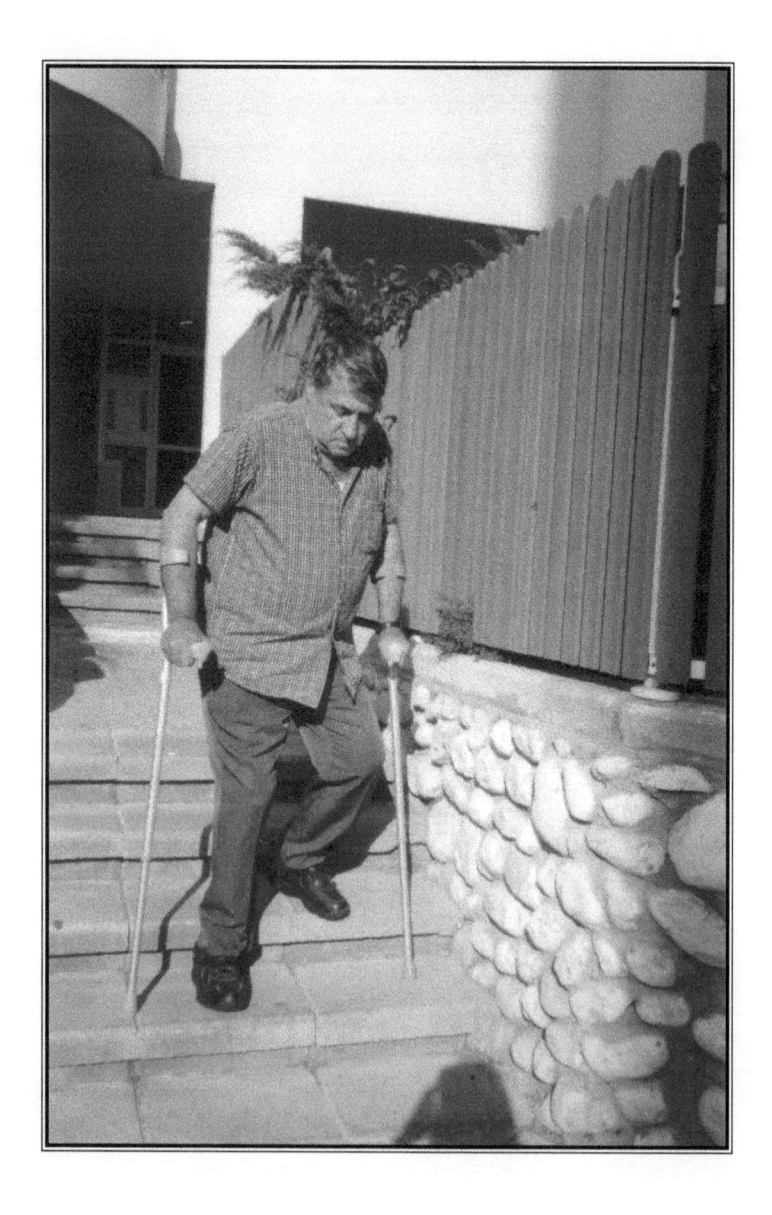

The new home; going for a walk in the new neighborhood.

The Will To Live

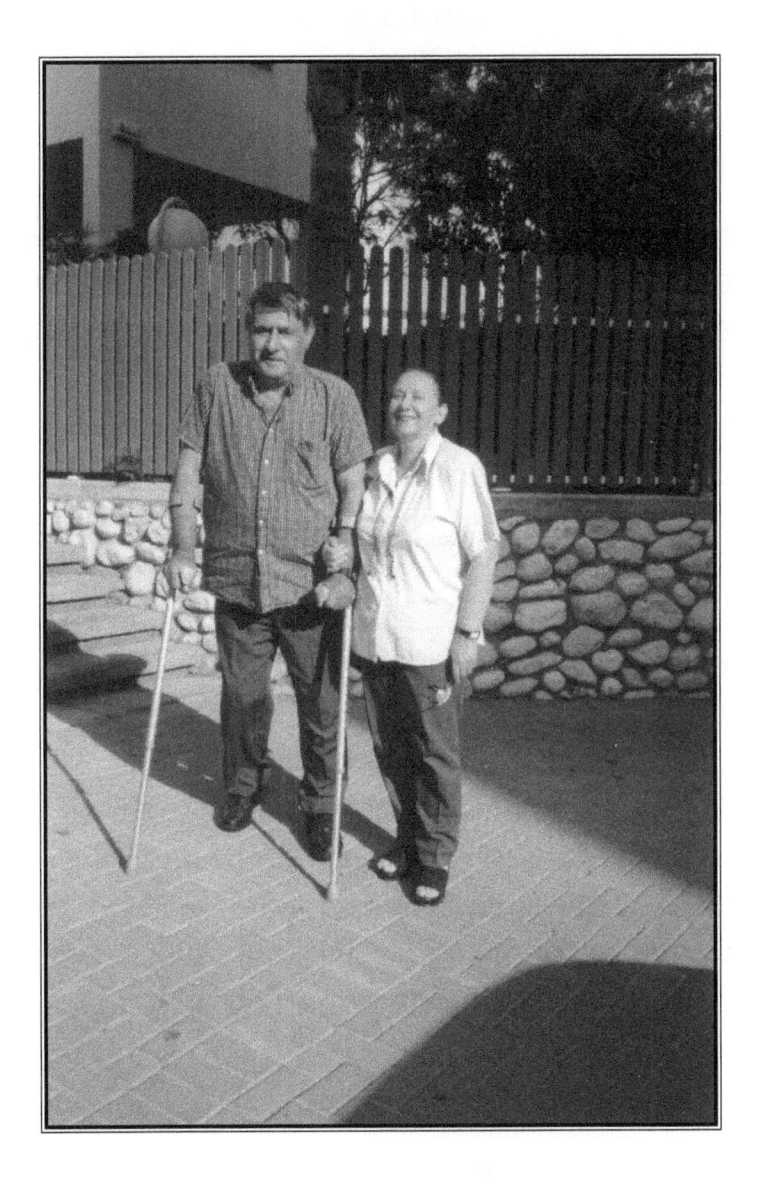

Arm in arm and heart to heart; my parents together on their new path.

Chapter 31
Today

Today, in 2008, my parents still go to the mall without a wheelchair. While my father has recovered from many of his injuries, his health is not what it was before the accident, and he returns to the hospital often, mostly due to reoccurring bouts of pneumonia. However, his will to live is strong, and although he is getting weaker (and not any younger!), my parents continue to enjoy their time in local coffee shops, having lots of fun together. When they are not "out on the town," they play cards, watch movies, and listen to music at home. They love to have visitors, and Dad occupies himself by reading books for many hours at a time. He also grows a nice little garden on the balcony of their home and is particularly proud of his "spicy peppers." They are still very dependent on each other, and when Mom goes grocery shopping, he calls her cell phone every half-hour! Even the shortest "parting" is hard on him.

* * *

Lots of events occurred in my personal life after Dad's accident. For one, I got divorced. Throughout the time Dad was in hospital, my husband was very supportive and took great care of the girls and our home while I was away. Although we are now parted, I will always be very grateful for that. Not long after my divorce, I fell in love with my soul-mate Edwin Orion Brownell, a concert-pianist, recording artist, and entertainer I had met at work. After a little over a year of dating we moved in together and have since been inseparable. As both of us love traveling and seeing our loved ones, we have gone to Israel annually to see my family and friends. Our latest visit was a very special occasion.

* * *

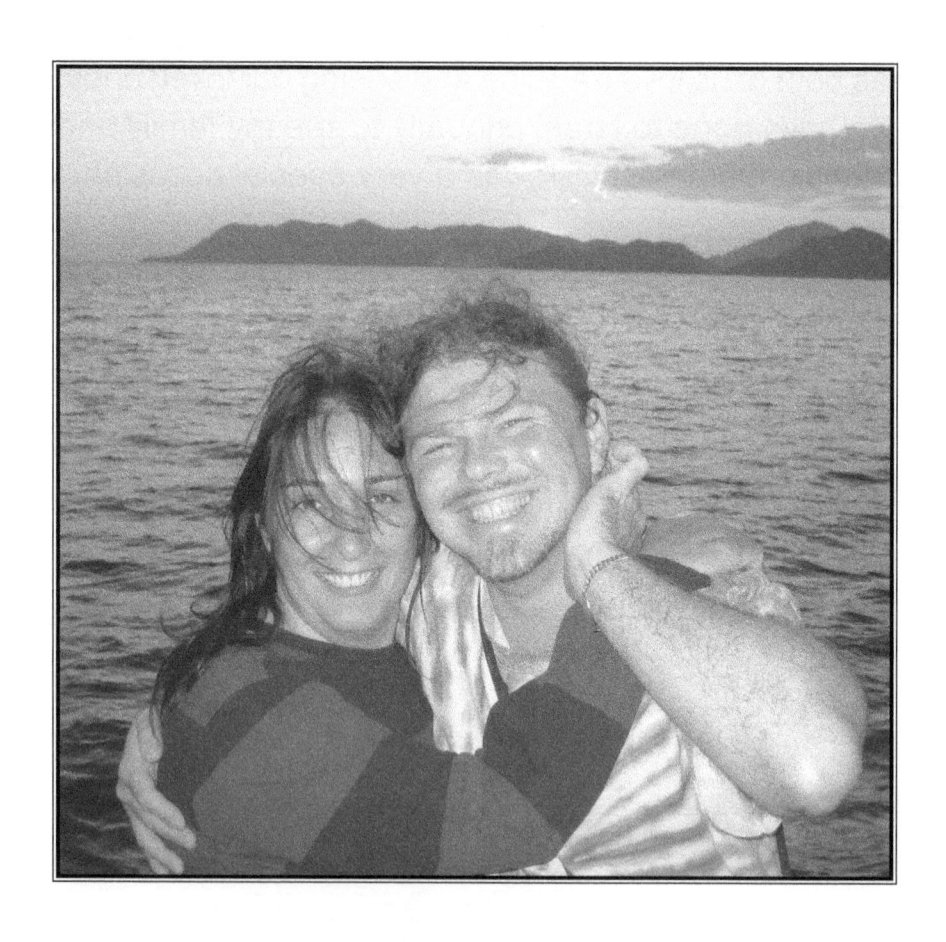

**Nechama with her sweetheart Edwin,
October 2008.**

In November, 2007, my parents celebrated their golden anniversary—fifty years together. The entire family was invited to spend this important and meaningful day with them in a restaurant in Rehovot across from Mom's and Dad's favorite mall.

It was an exciting event and everyone took part in the preparations.

I arrived in Israel early to make the necessary arrangements. I reserved the place, fixed the menu, and rented a piano to be delivered for the evening.

Yehuda brought the sound system, as his wife Aviva, is the owner of the biggest sound and light company in Israel. Their son Yaniv also helped, setting up the equipment prior to the event.

Finally, the work was done and the big evening had arrived. The family was almost all present, the tables were arranged beautifully, and the settings were elegant and very romantic.

At the entrance of the restaurant, my daughter Michal had set a table covered with a white tablecloth, flowers, and candles. On the table, she placed a magnificent Golden Anniversary Book which I had purchased in Canada. Everyone had managed to sign it before my parents arrived, just as we had planned.

On the wall, just behind the signing table, nobody could miss the two gorgeous pictures: my parents on their wedding day in Neve Monosson exactly fifty years ago, alongside a huge photo taken by Noam Moskovich, Michal's boyfriend. The wedding photo was enlarged and framed beautifully by Edwin and his mother. The more recent shot was taken when Noam (an art student at the prestigious Bezalel University in Jerusalem) and Michal had arranged a "photo day" about a week before the party. They took a series of pictures outside my parents' apartment, but no-one had seen the results until that evening. It was wonderful to see the two photos side by side. Although Mom and Dad looked different after a half-century, it was obvious that their love was unchanged and that their passion for each other was as full and as deep as ever. Michal and Noam had given them a very unique and heartfelt gift.

The stage was set, and all our family from Israel and abroad was waiting for the guests of honour to enter the room.

We had all lined up in two rows, and when my parents arrived we welcomed them with enthusiastic applause. Dad walked in slowly with his crutches, and Mom, as always, held his arm. My father looked very handsome wearing his tie and his best suit, and Mom was absolutely gorgeous with her elegant dress and a totally new haircut (it took me forever to convince her to try a new style!). They were very emotional as they were greeted by the family. After everyone had a chance to kiss them, we all sat down.

Edwin, as a concert pianist, took it upon himself to play with pride for my parents. As they first arrived and walked down the aisle with the family applauding, he played "*The Surik March,*" one of the two pieces he had composed especially for the celebration. After dinner, Edwin played everything from "*The Anniversary Waltz*" to "*Hava Nagila.*" Everyone danced; Yehuda and the youngest children got especially wild listening to the beautiful music. Halfway through the performance, Edwin congratulated my parents warmly while I translated. He dedicated the two original compositions that were written for this evening to them and then played the second: "*The Golden Dreams Waltz.*" Both works from his new double album were debuted that night. Edwin gave copies of his new CD to the entire family, but his greatest gift was the one he gave my parents: his love and his own enchanting music.

My sister-in-law Aviva wrote a gorgeous dedication to my parents about their devotion and love, and her daughter Sivan read it. Ayelet, Raffi's wife, followed in kind, speaking of the loyalty that my parents share for one another and the family. My aunt Chaviva also gave a moving speech about my parents, speaking of their love from the bottom of her heart. Yossi's wife Keren, a very creative craftswoman, carved a wonderful poem on a wooden plaque. She had lovingly embellished the beautiful words she had written with many intricate decorations.

The evening ended with a DVD that my daughter Shiri produced. Shiri couldn't come herself, but she and her boyfriend Ian Hermelin had put a lot of time and love into their gift. We played it on a large flat screen TV and everyone was treated to a slideshow of pictures showing the story of her grandparents' life together, from the day they started dating to their golden anniversary. She put music and captions to the pictures, and soon everyone without exception was wiping their eyes and blowing their noses, crying with happiness over a genuine love-story.

Oh, and myself. I prepared a surprise for my parents as well. They didn't have a clue about it. I presented them with the book *"The Will To Live."* It is a story about my mom and dad, two heroes; a love-story in which their **will to live** surpassed every obstacle in their way.

The Will To Live

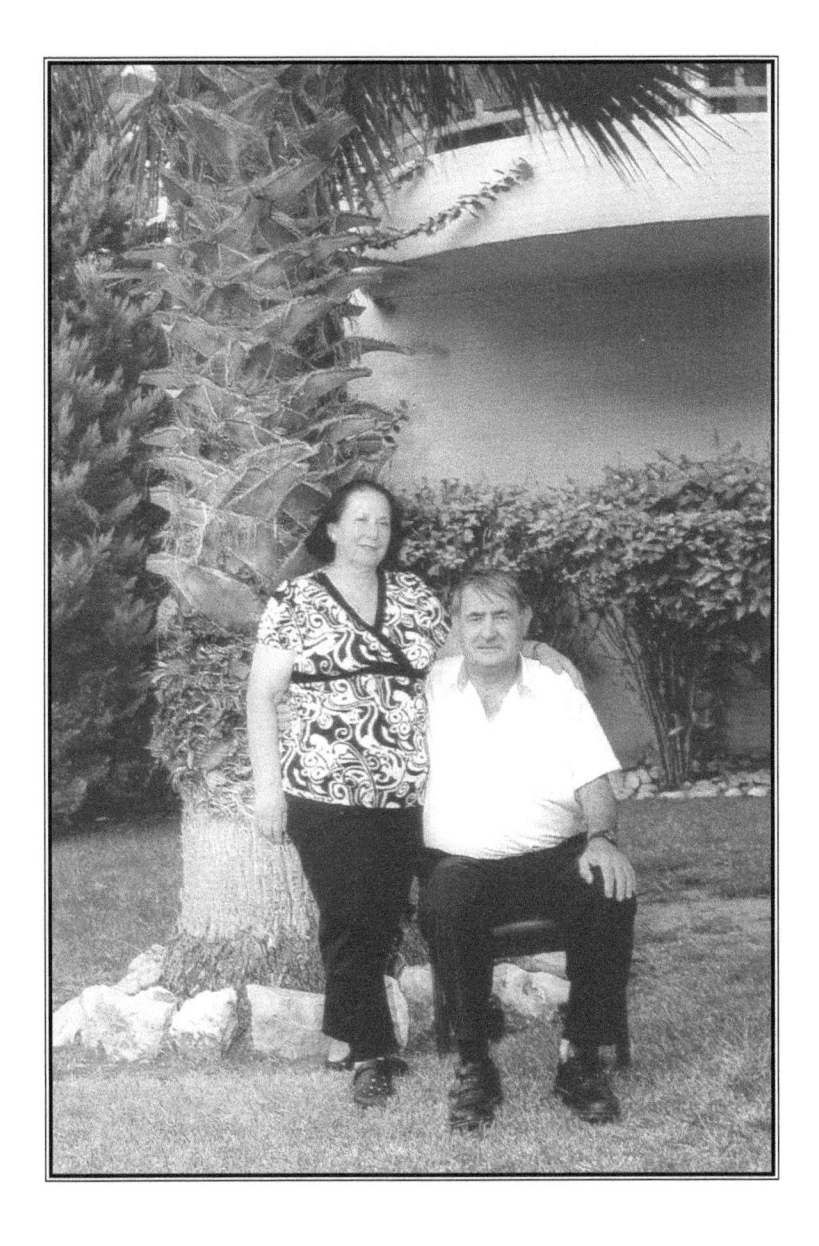

**The anniversary photo of the loving couple.
Photographer: Noam Moskovitch**

Lightning Source UK Ltd.
Milton Keynes UK
UKHW012019250521
384364UK00001B/40